Designing Your FACE

by Way Bandy

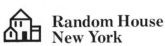
Random House
New York

Library of Congress Cataloging in Publication Data
Bandy, Way.
    Designing your face.
    1. Beauty, Personal.   2. Cosmetics.   I. Title.
RA778.B223   646.7′2   77-5962
ISBN 0-394-41908-1

Grateful acknowledgment is made to Dell Publishing Co., Inc. for permission to reprint the drawings by Way Bandy which appear in the chapter "Exercise." Reprinted from *Hairdo and Beauty*, June 1973. Copyright © 1973 by Hairdo Publishing Corporation.

Illustrations by Way Bandy

Manufactured in the United States of America
9 8 7 6 5 4 3

to
L.I. and Smudge

I wish to acknowledge with gratitude the generous assistance given to me by my editor, Susan Bolotin, and by my literary agent, Connie Clausen.

I offer special thanks to those who developed and produced **Designing Your Face** in its finished form: Rochelle Udell, book designer; Tony Wimpfheimer, managing editor; and Jan Tigner, production manager.

I was bored for most of my youth because I tried to do not only what was expected of me but also many other things I did not enjoy.

One day I realized that when you do something with your whole being simply because you love to do it, you experience life as it should be lived. It was then that I decided to be free and to do something I *loved* doing—creating beauty.

In 1969, when I began working professionally with cosmetics—something I really *love* doing—success and recognition came immediately. Since then, hundreds of people have contacted me, asking for help in learning to use cosmetics in the method and style I have created.

For those of you to whom I was not able to respond, perhaps this book will be of help and lead you to find freedom in your work and in your life.

Way Bandy

Contents

Introduction

Everyone admires beautiful bone structure, and everyone wishes to have beautiful skin. If you already have these assets, I will tell you how to enhance them. If you do not, I will show you how to use light, shadow, and color to give the illusion of good skin and good bones.

You must get to know your face—but really know it—inside and out. How can you improve the appearance of your facial bone structure if you are not aware of where your bones are, how they are shaped? This **knowing** is very difficult for some people. Most people look but do not **see**—especially one's own face.

We tend to **"retouch"** our expressions and reveal to our mirror only our best angles and most flattering illusions of reality, as seen through blurred vision and whatever other tricks we have at our disposal. Forget all that. Now you must face the **truth**—with no compromises!

Run to the nearest instant photo machine and take pictures of all the angles of your face that you can. Splurge! Spend a couple of bucks and get a good harsh look—you may have more assets than you expected. Also, have an enemy (not a sweet friend) take instant close-up photographs of your face from all angles.

Then study photographs of your entire body, standing and sitting, from every angle. Really try to be objective and regard these pictures as if they were of a stranger. Study the **lighting** in the photographs.

What is the source of light? How does it fall on the face? Where does the light come from when this stranger's face looks best? Top? Side? Bottom?

Now sit in front of a mirror and play with your face. Yes, use your hands to really **feel** your facial structure and skin quality and texture. Mentally remove your facial skin and look at the **skeletal structure** of your face and head.

Where do the bones protrude? Where do the bones indent? Where are the valleys and mountains of your personal facial landscape? Where do your teeth grow? Where and how do they attach to the bone? How do your teeth affect the sculpture of your face? Could an oral surgeon or orthodontist help the architecture of your teeth and face?

Do your bones tend to be angular or are they more rounded? Without your hair, how is you head shaped? What about your neck? Could improved posture through exercise training make your neck and head more elegant?

Now get acquainted with your skin. Where is your skin fleshy? Loose? Tight? Close to the bone? Porous? Rough? Smooth? Could a plastic surgeon redrape certain areas of the fabric of your skin and make your beauty life easier?

You must, through acute observation, arrive at an objective understanding of your skin coloring, texture and **drape**. Do you see your skin as more pink than yellow? Or vice versa? Ask friends if they would classify your skin coloring as either having pink undertones or yellow undertones. Do you have a ruddy, blotchy pigmentation or are you wonderfully creamy olive? On the street, try to classify broadly the skin undertones of strangers as red or yellow. Then refine your classifications to pink, rose, cream, yellow-olive, brown-red, yellow-brown, etc. Now try again, using this additional experience and knowledge, to classify your own skin undertone.

Is your skin texture fine-pored and thin so that you see tiny blue veins just underneath the surface, or is it as thick and pored as an orange peel? Or is it crinkled like fine tissue paper? Does it tend to fold from the nose to the corners of the mouth and at the jawline but have very few fine wrinkles? Or is it of medium thickness, rather tight on the bone, slightly irregular in texture?

One you **know** and **see** these characteristics of your skin color and texture you may wish you didn't (ignorance *is* bliss). However, this kind of brutal analysis is necessary in order to know where and how you need to improve your appearance cosmetically.

Now, if you haven't taken to your bed in despair, go for a walk down the street and look at the faces of others. Ask the same questions—what a revelation! It is like an art appreciation course in which you analyze a painting and really see it for the first time after having known it for years. As a matter of fact, you should also study famous portraits by master painters. Try to see the arrangement of light and shadow that gives the illusion of valleys and mountains to a face. What colors and textures seem to make the skin look thick and loose and which ones give the impression of thin, taut, translucent skin? And of normal, healthy, firm skin?

With all this analysis you will begin to recognize and appreciate the individuality of human faces; to see the beauty in some so-called flaws; to understand how spirit and personality vitalize expression; to realize that for centuries good skin and good bones have passed for great beauty; to know that classical elegance of facial beauty transcends style, fashion, whim.

You will also begin to understand from your analysis of the human face why I refer to the finished product, after one uses cosmetics to create the illusion of beautiful skin and bones, as a SCULPTURE-PORTRAIT. Not only does one paint color onto the face but also one seems to sculpt better bones with light and dark tones.

After you completely understand all your negative and positive facial qualities and have mastered this method of creating beauty through illusion, I hope that you always approach yourself as the greatest of beauties—because then you will have the means to make it so.

Although there are few ironclad rules involved in this method of creating the illusion of beauty using cosmetics, there is a definite pattern and technique of application which one must master before kicking over the traces. Just as one must learn to sketch and draw with pencil or charcoal before having a free hand at watercolors and oils, so must one learn the basic design for using cosmetics to paint a face before experimenting with advanced techniques of beauty through illusion.

Obviously, these techniques apply to all skin colorations from the lightest blond Swede to the darkest black Ethiopian. It is all a matter of light, dark, and color as they apply to your skin tones.

The FACE DESIGNS given here are timeless and ageless. You are working with your individual skin texture and color and with your unique bone structure. Whether you are very young or very old is irrelevant. Use as many or as few of these cosmetic techniques as you feel comfortable with. Generally speaking, as one gets older, **less** is **more**.

Nothing is more attractive to me than the person who has the spirit and intelligence to strive for even more individuality—the exaggerated flaw that signifies style, chic. I do suggest that you develop an awareness of skin and bones and master the basic application techniques necessary to create a SCULPTURE-PORTRAIT, but the last thing I wish to do with this presentation of my patterns and techniques of application is to set limitations on individuality. The very nature of using one's own skin and bones as a guide rather than trying to meet an impossible ideal suggests, I hope, my fond regard for the eccentric conceit that sets each of us apart as unique beings.

Equipment

Let us get right to the heart of the matter—equipment to get started. You do not need a vast array of colors and textures, but you do need several specific items. Do not waste time asking why at this point—just try to learn as much about as many of these things as possible. (Refer to the color insert in this book to match shades when shopping.) After you are beautiful you can get into **why**—if you are still interested.

Fluids

—protective skin lotion

(All moisturizers are not "protective." Some evaporate so quickly that they actually cause dryness. A **protective** skin lotion leaves a slight film on the skin that may help to retain some moisture at the skin surface—and may possibly block out some pollutants from the atmosphere. Read the list of ingredients!

If there is any ingredient you do not know, don't put the moisturizer on your face until you find out what that ingredient is and what it may do for or against the health of your skin. You may find an effective product in a health food store that proudly lists the simple, natural ingredients.)

—opaque white liquid foundation

(Though this product should be thin, watery and chalk-white, it should give opaque coverage.)

—light beige liquid foundation
—medium beige liquid foundation
—dark beige liquid foundation
—transparent red-colored fluid
—transparent peach-colored fluid
—transparent bronze-colored fluid
—skin freshener or distilled water

(The skin freshener you choose should be very mild—preferably without alcohol and/or other harsh chemicals.)

(These fluids should ideally be **transparent;** however, since you may not find them easily, you may have to settle for **translucent** washes of color that are readily available from several cosmetic companies.)

Creams
—medium-toned fleshy warm brown shadow cream (**dark 1**)
—dark-toned greyed earth-brown shadow cream (**dark 2**)
—light neutral beige creamy paste (**light**)

(None of these foundations should contain red, orange, pink, or grey pigments that are obvious either in the container or when tested on the skin. The colors should be truly neutral beiges.)

—red creamy paste (**color glow**)
—clear, shiny lip gloss

Pencils
—charcoal medium-grey eyeliner pencil
—black eye liner pencil
—beige-blond eyebrow pencil
—No. 6325 artist pencil
—auburn (or reddish-brown) pencil

Powder
—translucent, no-color baby talcum

Tools

—black brush-wand mascara

—eyelash curler

—three (3) soft, fluffy, washable powder brushes

—eyebrow brush

—eyelash brush and/or comb

—square-tipped lip brush

—slant-tipped tweezer

—sharpener for cosmetic pencils

—two or three soft, flat, square-tipped brushes for applications of **light**, **dark 1**, **dark 2**

Ideally, the listed equipment products should not contain iridescent ingredients; they should have transparent or translucent flat finishes when applied to the skin.

This may seem a formidable list of equipment for one face, but do not despair—there is more later! And think of all the mounds of junk cosmetics you have stashed right now. Actually, these listed items are all things you will use regularly.

When you have learned to shape and color your face with these products, you will never again worry about what to buy—you will **know**—and probably more than the salesperson behind the counter.

Although you may not think so at this point, I plan to simplify your beauty life—not complicate it. Patience!

Fluids

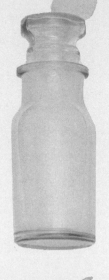

protective
skin
lotion

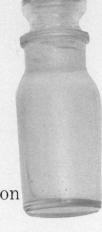

opaque
white
liquid
foundation

skin
freshener
or
distilled
water

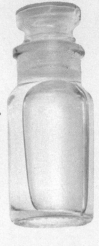

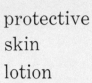

light
beige
liquid
foundation

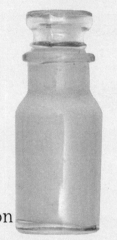

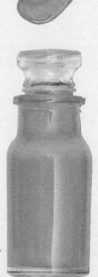

medium
beige
liquid
foundation

dark
beige
liquid
foundation

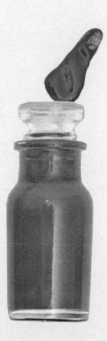

transparent
red-colored
fluid

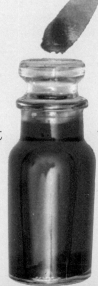

transparent
peach-colored
fluid

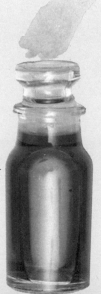

transparent
bronze-colored
fluid

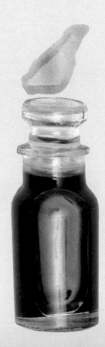

Powder

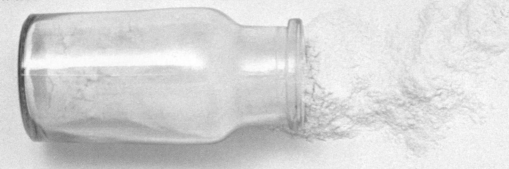

translucent, no-color baby talcum

Pencils

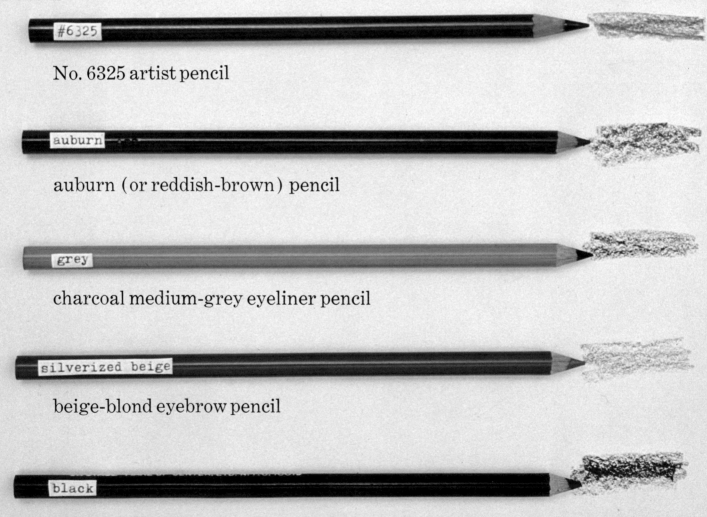

#6325

No. 6325 artist pencil

auburn

auburn (or reddish-brown) pencil

grey

charcoal medium-grey eyeliner pencil

silverized beige

beige-blond eyebrow pencil

black

black eye liner pencil

Creams

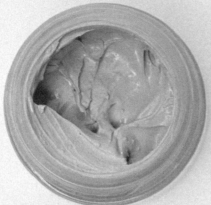

light neutral
beige creamy paste
(**light**)

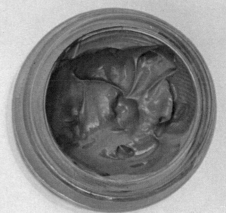

dark beige
creamy paste
(**to be used as light on
very dark skin**)

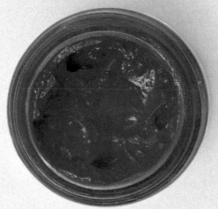

red creamy paste
(**color glow**)

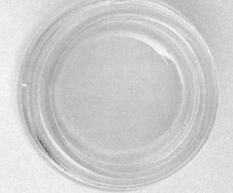

clear, shiny
lip gloss

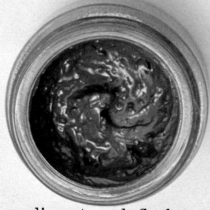

medium-toned fleshy
warm brown
shadow cream
(**dark 1**)

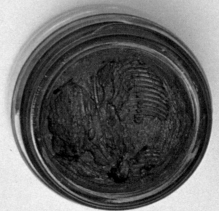

dark-toned greyed
earth-brown
shadow cream
(**dark 2**)

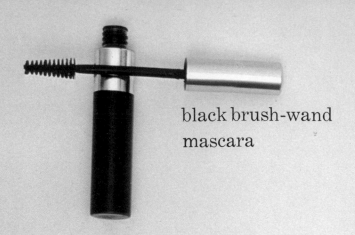

black brush-wand
mascara

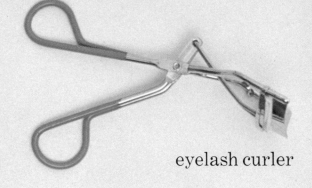

eyelash curler

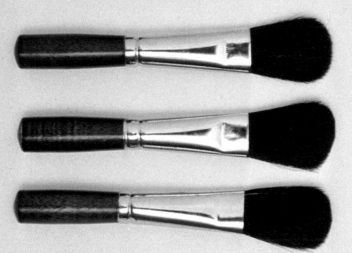

three (3) soft, fluffy, washable
powder brushes

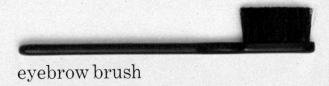

eyelash brush and/or comb

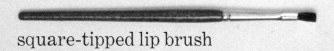

eyebrow brush

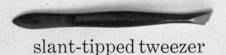

square-tipped lip brush

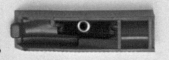

slant-tipped tweezer

two or three soft, flat, square-tipped
brushes for applications of **light,
dark 1, dark 2**

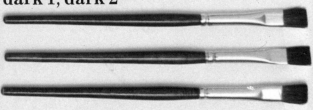

sharpener for
cosmetic pencils

Worktable

When you have collected your equipment you must then arrange a worktable either where the lighting is suitable or where you can make the lighting suitable.

Sit about six feet from a window with natural daylight streaming in toward your face. Your worktable should be in front of you so that you will be looking into the mirror. This setup is ideal, but if it is neither feasible nor comfortable for you, you may try this alternative: Place your worktable about eight feet from the window so that you are sitting with your back to the window. The daylight will then come over your shoulder and reflect into the mirror, lighting your face.

Artificial lighting should come from the sides at eye level—not from above or from below. The light bulbs should be frosted to reduce glare, and definitely incandescent rather than fluorescent. Both distort color, but incandescent does so in your favor, while fluorescent works against you —besides draining your energy through excess radiation! You should also have a hand mirror with one side that magnifies.

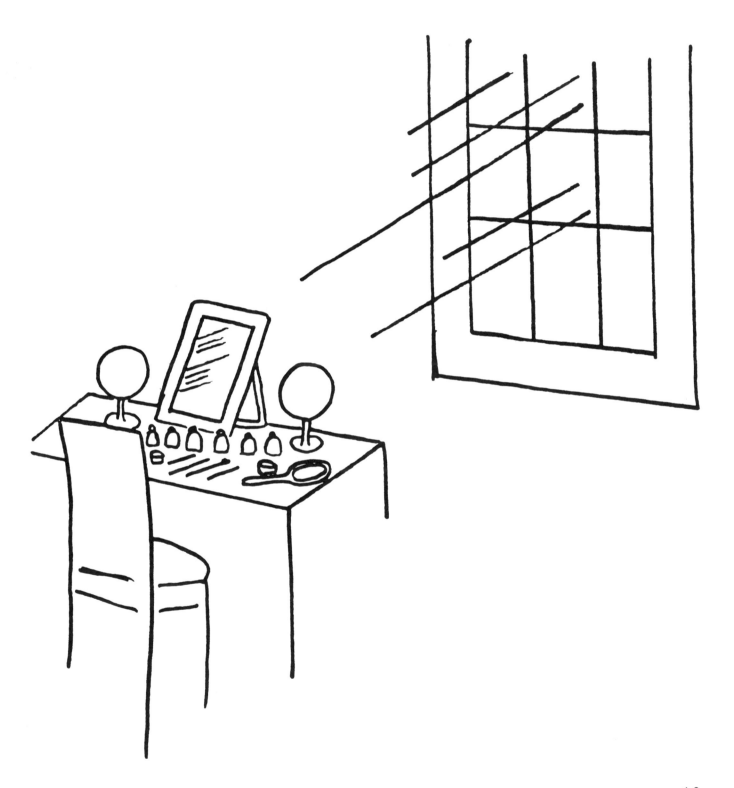

Eyebrows

Eyebrows can make or break a face. In my opinion there should be more rules concerning eyebrows than any other part of the face. Once you are aware of the correct way to shape, groom, and color eyebrows you will see that many mistakes are made in attempting to beautify the eyebrows.

Aesthetically speaking, the eyebrow is a frame for the eye. When considering a frame for a picture, one thinks of complementing and emphasizing the shape, color, proportion, and mood of the picture being framed. One would not select a frame whose shape or color would conquer the picture but, rather, one that would subtly enhance the picture it surrounds. The same theory applies to eyebrows.

Procedure

1. Sit and look directly into your mirror at the shape of your top lid along the line where your lashes grow.

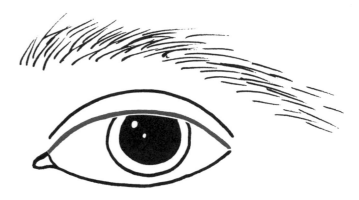

2. Now (with your eyes looking directly into your mirror) consider this **lashline** as a pencil mark drawn onto a blank piece of paper. This shape of your very individual lashline will serve as the guide for shaping, if necessary, your eyebrow line. Your lashline may be a very slight semicircle ; or it may be a very arched one ; or it may go up at the outside ; or down . Whatever the shape, it will be yours alone and like no one else's.

3. You should make the **undercurve** of your eyebrow conform in shape to the curve of your top lashline when the eye is looking directly into your mirror. Some plucking of stray hairs with tweezers will probably be necessary to create the desired eyebrow shape. I find a slant-tipped tweezer, rather than a pointed, round, or square-tipped one, to be the easiest to work with.

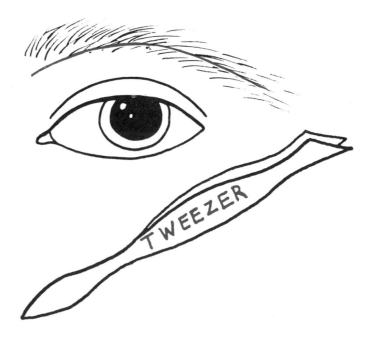

4. The next question that arises is where to begin the eyebrow and where to end it? The eyebrow should begin directly above the very inside corner of the eye and it should fade to a gradually tapered end beyond the outside corner of the eye at no definite, abrupt point. One should not be aware of the ending of the eyebrow —it should be a fade-out somewhere beyond the outside corner of the eye.

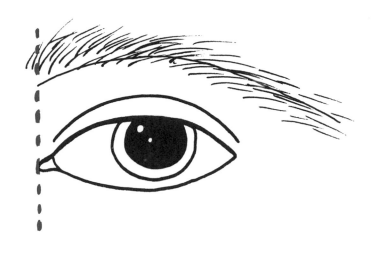

5. With a slant-tipped tweezer, remove any eyebrow hairs that grow outside the desired curve under the brows or between the brows. Be careful not to tweeze so precisely that either the undercurve or the inside corner of the brow has an unnaturally sharp, definite edge. Hairs grow irregularly, and you should tweeze a slightly irregular shape that lacks total precision so that it is not obvious that the eyebrow has been shaped by tweezing. The brow should not be tweezed into a curved line à la Dietrich—a lady for whom I have total admiration, but who was always under carefully controlled lighting that showed her best angles. (With a little awareness of the aesthetics of balance

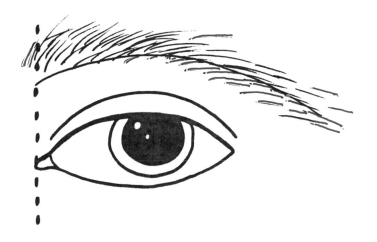

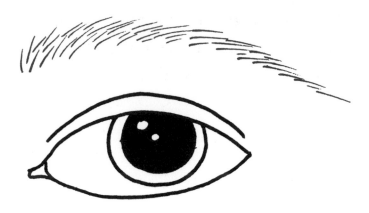

and proportion, some of our other great beauties from the silver screen could have been even more extraordinary.)

6. Unless you have white, light grey, or very blond hair, the color of your eyebrows should be a few shades lighter than your hair color. Would one ever put a much darker frame on a light picture unless one wished to call attention to the frame itself?

It may be necessary to lighten by bleaching eyebrows that are much darker than your hair color. You may use a facial hair bleach and leave it on the eyebrows **not more than two minutes.** Better to **underbleach** and have to do it again for a few seconds than to leave the bleach on too long and suddenly have bright orange eyebrows. Remember, you are bleaching only to cut the darkness of the hairs of the eyebrows. Only a tone or two lighter makes a terrific difference when you stand back from your mirror and look at your entire face and head.

I wish to include all the information about eyebrows in this chapter; therefore, even though you will use Step 7 later, near the end of the chapter on eyes, the following information about coloring and shaping the eyebrows with pencils is given here.

7. There is one eyebrow pencil color that, oddly enough, I have found to be so versatile that it is suitable for almost all eyebrows. It is a beige-blond color that is often referred to as **silverized beige.** It is so neutral a beige that one almost cannot apply it too darkly.

For very dark brows, using a No. 6325 artist pencil is an old trick used by many actresses and models for shaping eyebrows. Perhaps you could try a mixture of the two pencils—silverized beige and No. 6325.

A brow pencil should be very sharp so that you are able to simulate tiny hairs growing. Always apply with feather strokes in the upward and outward direction that the brow hairs grow. Then use an eyebrow brush (or child's toothbrush) to soften your pencil strokes and blend them with the real hairs. You should finish with a soft, subtle brow shape that is blended enough to trick the viewer's eye into assuming that your eyebrow grew that way naturally.

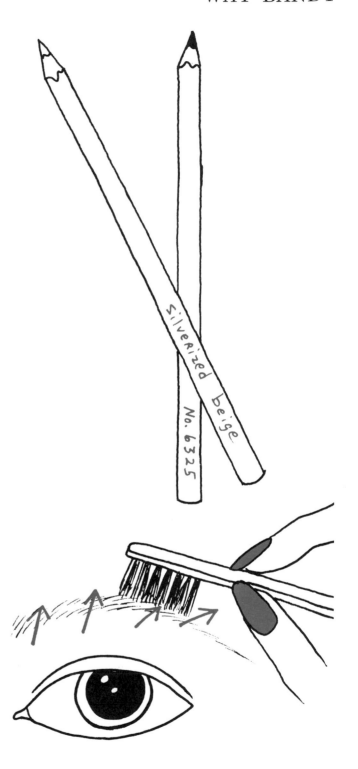

Complexion Prime Coat

Regardless of your skin undertones or texture, you must begin your personal SCULPTURE-PORTRAIT by creating a neutrally colored beige-tone canvas with as smooth and fine a texture as possible. This first step in creating the illusion of beautiful skin is literally the foundation on which your face is built. One should spend as much time and effort to perfect this process as one does later on shaping and enlarging the eyes. I call this first step applying the **complexion prime coat.** It should accomplish four things:

- coverage
- color
- glow
- the illusion of smooth skin texture

16

Procedure

Here is the procedure for mixing the formula that suits your complexion:

1. Select the following items from your worktable
—one beige liquid foundation that is nearest to your overall skin color (light, medium, or dark beige)
—one opaque white liquid foundation
—one mild skin freshener or distilled water
—one protective skin lotion
—(if you have red undertones) one transparent bronze fluid
—(if you have yellow undertones) one transparent red fluid

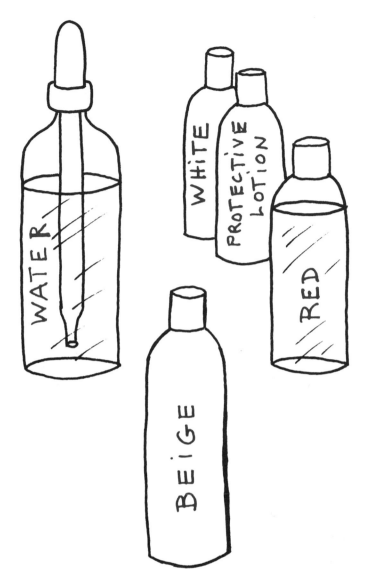

2. The goal of mixing these five ingredients is to give the impression of color without coverage. This will require some experimentation and practice on your part. You may have to vary the amounts of each ingredient from day to day depending on changes in your skin color and condition. However, here is a basic formula with which to begin.

Recipe

Use the palm of your left hand as a mixing bowl (your right palm if you are left-handed) and start with this mixture:

—one nickel-sized drop of beige liquid foundation (for coverage)

—one pea-sized drop of opaque white liquid foundation (for neutralization)

—one nickel-sized drop of transparent colored fluid (red or bronze depending on your skin undertone) for glow

—two pea-sized drops of protective skin lotion (for texture)

—one quarter-sized drop of skin freshener or distilled water (for thinning the mixture to avoid opaque coverage)

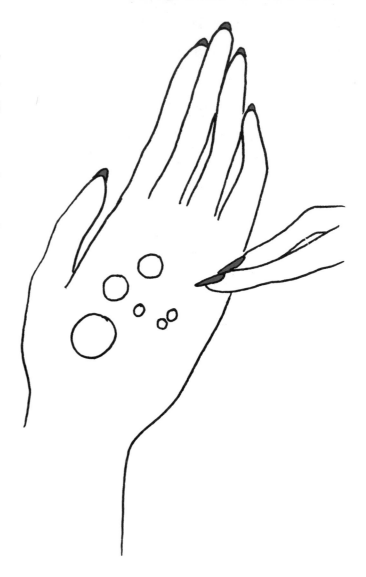

3. Use a fingertip to mix these five ingredients until they combine into one thin, watery, flesh-colored fluid—the **complexion prime coat**. (I shall refer to it by using the abbreviation "CPC.")

4. Apply the CPC with fingertips to the entire face and blend downward onto the neck and back over the ears —this is the prime coat for your personal sculpture-portrait. As you apply, think of blending the CPC *into* the skin rather than *onto* the skin, and you will find yourself using the fingertips quite differently.

5. When the first coat of CPC is on, your skin should begin to look smoother, more glowing and more evenly colored. Where you need more coverage apply one or two or even three more coats of the thin fluid CPC. I have discovered that many thin coats give a much more realistic skin appearance than one thick, heavy, opaque coat of foundation. But apply these extra coats of CPC only where you need them for more coverage.

It is a must that you cover your entire face with CPC including over and under the eyes and right up to the hair line. You are attempting to create a new skin surface—a canvas to paint on. So get it on smoothly, evenly, and beautifully.

Obviously, you will always have at hand on your worktable the colors you need for your seasonal skin-color changes. If you have a tan from the sun, just add a bit more bronze fluid and skip the white foundation in your CPC mixture.

If you have a sun tan and your ordinarily light or medium skin is darker than usual

Recipe
—one nickel-sized drop of beige liquid foundation
—one quarter-sized drop of bronze transparent fluid
—two pea-sized drops of protective skin lotion
—one quarter-sized drop of skin freshener or distilled water

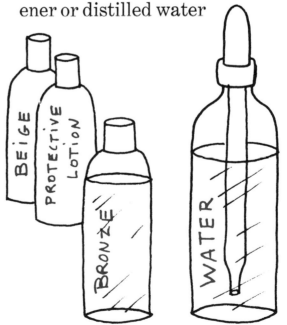

On the other hand, if you are winter-pale, add more white liquid foundation and use a lighter beige liquid foundation in your CPC mixture.

Recipe
For winter-pale skin
—one nickel-sized drop of light beige liquid foundation
—two pea-sized drops of opaque white liquid foundation
—one nickel-sized drop of transparent colored fluid (red or bronze or peach)
—two pea-sized drops of protective skin lotion
—one quarter-sized drop of skin freshener or distilled water

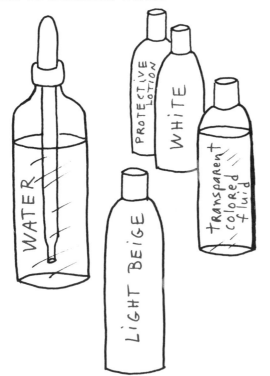

Brighten a yellowish sun tan by adding more red fluid, and thin the CPC even more than usual with skin freshener or distilled water to allow the glow of sun-warmed skin to show through. Or mix just the peach transparent fluid in equal parts with the bronze transparent fluid, thin with protective skin lotion, and work the mixture into the skin for a sunny, healthy-looking glow any time of year.

Recipe
For a sunny, healthy-looking glow any time of year
—one nickel-sized drop of peach transparent fluid
—one nickel-sized drop of bronze transparent fluid
—one nickel-sized drop of protective skin lotion

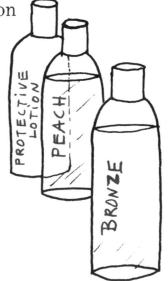

If your skin is very dark beige or dark brown you will be more likely to have yellow undertones rather than red. However, there are exceptions, and you must diligently analyze and observe (as directed earlier in this book) to determine if your skin is more red or more yellow in colortone.

You may have to experiment with the red transparent fluid and with the bronze transparent fluid (classified as the more yellow of the transparent fluids from your worktable) to help you to determine which is more complimentary to your particular skin color.

After you have made your decision as to which transparent fluid you will use, then mix a basic formula omitting any opaque white liquid foundation (which tends to make very dark skins have a grey or ashen appearance).

Recipe

For very dark beige or very dark brown skin colorations

—one nickel-sized drop of dark beige liquid foundation

—two nickel-sized drops of transparent colored fluid (red or bronze depending on your skin undertone)

—two pea-sized drops of protective skin lotion

—one quarter-sized drop of skin freshener or distilled water

Mix in the palm of your hand and apply to the entire face and blend slightly down onto the neck.

This CPC recipe is the basic starting formula. Of course, you will make changes in the amounts used as you experiment with your coloring.

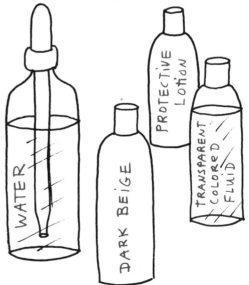

Contouring with Light

If one applies a very light beige-colored thin paste or crayon to the skin, that area where it is placed seems to come forward, stand out from the face, be highlighted—lifted out of shadow. If you have learned your face well, you will know where the unattractive valleys are—those valleys or indentations that cause a **shadow area** that adds age to the appearance of the face. At the bottom of these indentations is where you will place the light beige-colored thin paste. I call this product **light** because it does seem to bring light to deep, shadowed valleys.

The **light** product you choose should be a few shades lighter than your CPC but not so light that it appears white, opaque, and chalky. Perhaps you will have to mix with a small spatula two or three colors of **light** in a jar to arrive at one that suits you exactly.

Procedure

Here are the valleys you may need to improve with an application of **light:**

1. Under the eyes along the base of the area where one might develop a loose bag or pouch in the aging process.

The area directly under the eye, near the lower lashes, often protrudes. By applying **light** there the protrusion or puffiness would be exaggerated, so avoid that area.

2. In the socket or small but often very deep valley, just between the edge of the bridge of the nose and the inside corner of the eye.

3. In the crease around the outer edges of the nostrils and along the folds that run diagonally from the crease of the nostrils to the outside corners of the mouth.

Light must be placed only at the very bottom of these valleys—not up on the edge of the cliff; otherwise, this area will look puffy and protruding.

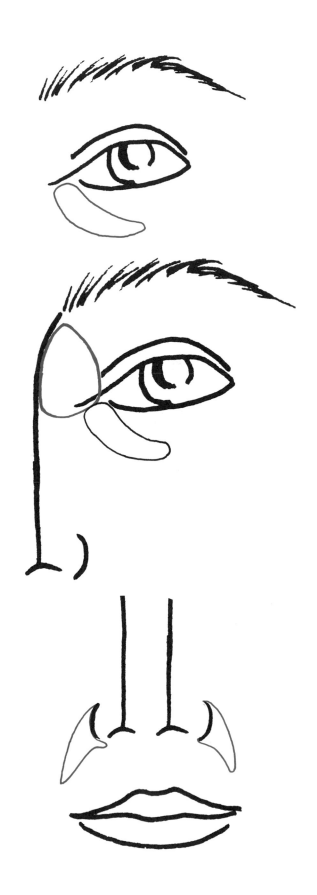

23

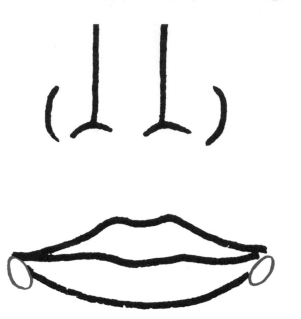

4. Just below the outside corners of the mouth, if a small pocket or valley exists there.

You may apply **light** with a small, flat, square-tipped brush or with a fingertip. I like to use my hands as much as possible to avoid so many tools of application; however, you may work easier with a brush.

Once you have applied the **light** in the proper areas, you must use your fingertips for blending. **Do not rub** or blend with long, eager strokes. If you do so, you will move the **light** away from the very specific areas of placement. Instead, use a fingertip to **touch and press** (as if you were blotting) the **light** into the skin. Keep a tissue near to constantly clean your fingertips, as the warmth of your skin tends to melt the **light** and your finger will lift away any excess of the product. This **touch and press** technique is crucial to the sculpting and molding of the face. Since it is one of the keys to a successful SCULPTURE-POR-TRAIT and will be used repeatedly further along in these lessons, learn it well now! As you touch and press the **light** you will see it blend into the CPC so that you do not see edges definitely; rather, the **light** will gradually, imperceptibly become part of the CPC.

5.   To build a higher cheekbone, place **light** in this manner on the top of the cheekbone: Consider that your cheekbone is a ledge protruding from a building. It has a top running at a slight diagonal from the outside corner of the eye directly outward to the hairline at the base of the temple. Now look directly into your mirror and mentally sketch an **imaginary dotted line** vertically from the outside corner of the eye straight up and down.

Disregard the mountains and valleys (or planes) of your bone and skin structure and try to visualize your whole face as a **flat** plane—a piece of paper on which you can sketch a straight line. This **imaginary dotted line** will be your guide not only for placement of **light** on the cheekbone but also for other steps in building your bone structure—so get this set in your head now.

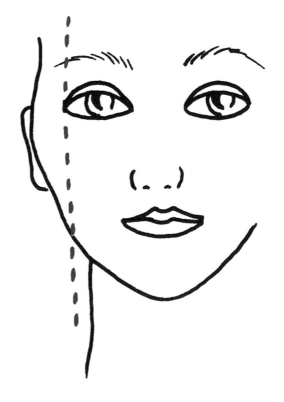

25

This concept may seem slightly complicated if you are skimming through this book, but if you have become familiar with your facial skin and bones through practical application of the preceding instructions, the imaginary line should be a snap.

6. Sketch straight down with **light** (using a brush, a fingertip, or a crayon if your **light** is in stick form) from the outside corner of the eye about one-half inch to the highest point of the cheekbone—then a line straight from eye corner to hairline.

7. Then sketch a straight line diagonally across the ridge of the cheekbone to close the triangle.

8. Fill in this triangular outline with **light** and use the **touch and press** method to blend this entire shape into nothingness so that no edges are apparent.

From a profile point of view the triangular shape should look like this sketch.

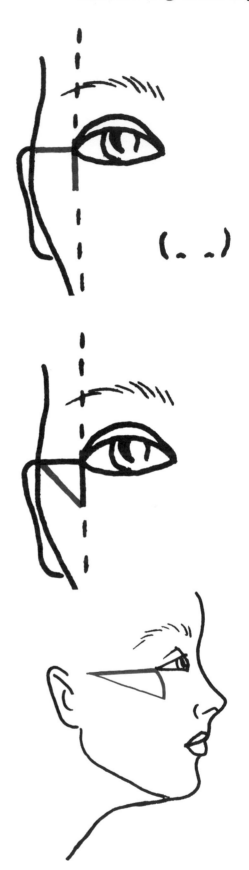

Contouring with Dark

On certain unattractive mountains of your facial landscape you can apply dark tones of shadow cream to give the illusion of a flatter mountain or even, in some cases, a valley. Shadow cream (which I refer to here as **dark**) may also be used to make an area next to it seem to protrude or come forward more dramatically. These areas usually need **dark:**

—the orbital bone that protrudes beneath the eyebrow
—the sides of the nose—particularly at the bridge and sometimes across the flare of the nostrils—and under the tip end of the nose
—under the ledge of the cheekbones
—under the tip of the chin and along the jawbone

The **dark** products used should be of two different tonalities. One should be a **fleshy, warm brown.** The other should be a **cool greyed earth-brown.** Henceforth, these products will be referred to by the abbreviations **dark 1** and **dark 2.**

Real shadows have many depths of tone ranging from light to dark and in range of coloration from warm to cool. Therefore, in order to create the illusion of a natural shadow one must use a minimum of two tones.

If you are to be photographed or if you are going out for an evening where there will be very soft lighting, you may wish to shadow the sides of your nose to simulate a better proportion of nose to entire face or just to add an element of refinement and balance to your SCULPTURE-POR-TRAIT.

Procedure

1. Look straight into your mirror and visualize your nostrils as two horizontal lines drawn onto a flat surface. Your nostrils may be small housetops ∧ ∧ or inverted semi-circles ⌒ ⌒, but you must realize them as more horizontal —— than vertical | . Now locate the exact center of each short horizontal line which represents a nostril.

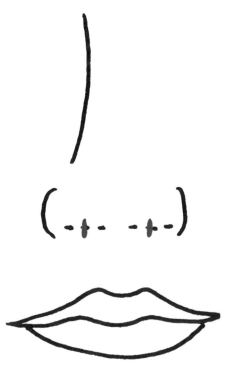

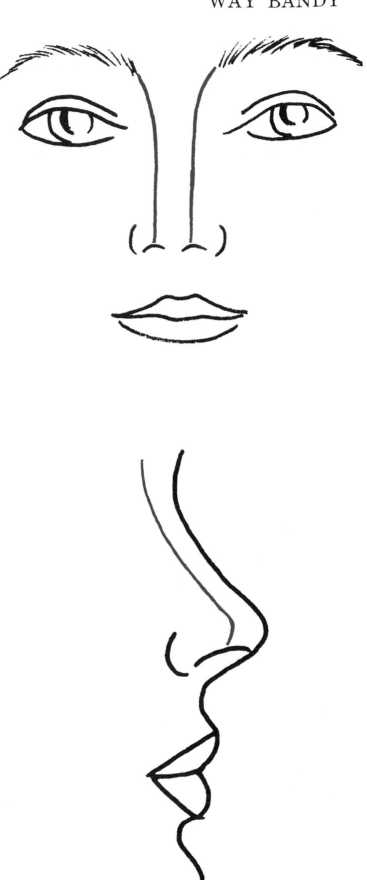

2. These center marks will be your guides for drawing **dark 1** shadow cream with a fine brush or your fingertip **vertical parallel lines** straight up the sides of the nose to the bridge of the nose, then curving the lines upward and outward to join the beginning of the eyebrows.

It is imperative that you continue to look straight into your mirror and even more important that you visualize your nose area as a flat plane like a piece of paper as you draw **straight vertical lines.** The nose is usually a series of slightly irregular planes (valleys and mountains) and different on each side. You may have a bump on one side and an indentation on the other. Your job is to mentally erase these irregularities and to visualize them as flat so that your vertical lines are **straight** and **parallel.**

When you view your work in profile you may be quite surprised that your straight lines seem to be curved. That is because of the irregular planes that you have "straightened" from a frontal view.

29

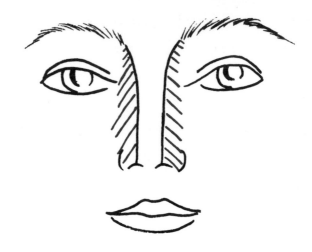

3. Using a delicate touch of your fingertip and being extremely careful not to move any of the **dark 1** shadow cream **inside** your parallel lines, blend the **dark 1** by **touching and pressing** with a slight movement outward onto the sides of the nose and the flare of the nostrils. The outer edges of the shadow-cream area should not be apparent but should blend (like all other edges in your SCULPTURE-POR-TRAIT) imperceptibly into nothing-ness.

4. You may give the illusion of shortening the nose slightly by applying shadow cream under the very tip of the nose. First sketch across the tip horizontally between the two vertical lines. This connecting line should be placed exactly at the point where the tip of the nose starts sloping back-ward and downward toward the upper-lip area. **Touch and press** to blend the **dark 1** shadow cream under the tip of the nose.

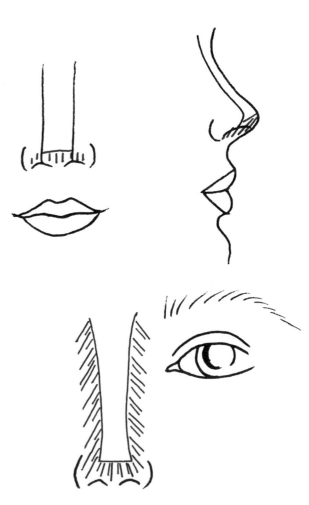

5. If you want to test your profi-ciency, you may now sketch the nar-rowest possible line of **dark 2** shadow cream along the inside edge of the

30

vertical parallel lines on the nose to create depth of shadow.

Please do not ever attempt this for the street or daylight. Even the first step of nose shading with **dark 1** should be attempted for street wear only by the most expert of artists. Creating artificial shadows to shape and refine the nose should be reserved only for very soft evening lighting or for professional use. Otherwise, you may appear to have a dirty nose —even with the most careful blending.

Now back to the cheekbone. Again, visualize the cheekbone as a ledge protruding from a building. A ledge has a top, a side, and a bottom. So does a cheekbone.

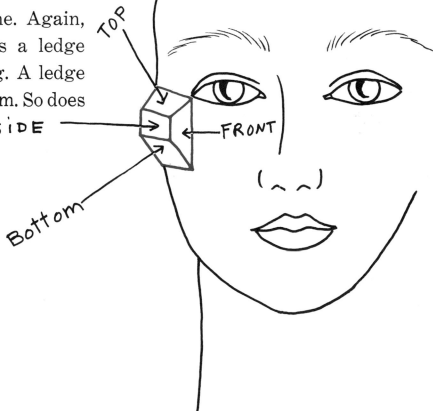

We have already discussed the top of the ledge in the **light** lesson. Now let us focus on the structure of what I consider to be about the most beautiful bone in the human face—the cheekbone. Touch the outside corner of your right eye with the tip of your right index finger. Then rest the length of that finger along the top ledge of the cheekbone base to the hairline at the base of the temple area. Do you begin to be aware of the cheekbone ledge? Now slightly **roll** the finger downward onto the side of the cheekbone plane; slide the same index finger downward and it will move under the bottom plane of the cheekbone ledge. Repeat the same procedure with the left index finger on the left cheekbone.

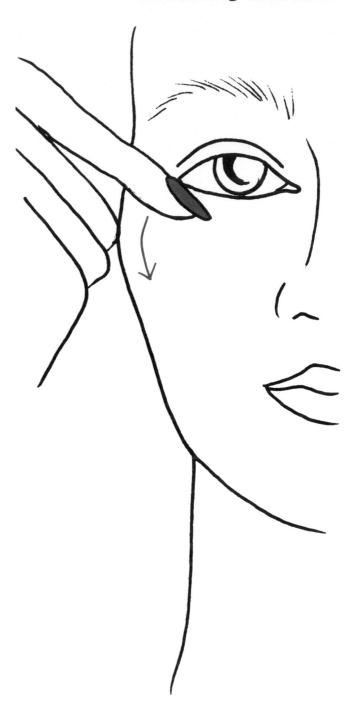

Try this same procedure on a friend's cheekbones. Although a ledge on a building has sharp edges and the ledge of your cheekbone has more rounded edges, I think you can now begin to grasp the similarity. This kind of familiarity with the structure of your face is necessary in order to realize the transformation (using cosmetics) of aesthetically unattractive or ordinary skin and bones into a SCULPTURE-PORTRAIT of extraordinary physical beauty.

Procedure

1. Starting underneath the bottom front edge of the cheekbone ledge (at the imaginary dotted line running vertically from the outside corner of the eye downward toward the jaw line, as illustrated), sketch the **dark 1** shadow cream **underneath** the cheekbone back to the ear or wherever your cheekbone joins the edge of your face.

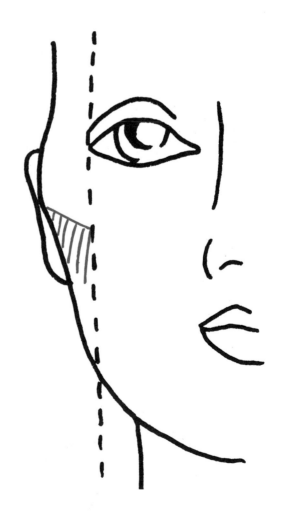

2.   Using the **touch and press** method and continually cleaning your fingertip on a tissue to remove excess shadow cream, blend the approximately half-inch-wide band of **dark 1** shadow cream downward and backward into an almost imperceptible edge.

3.   Exactly under the cheekbone **at the very edge** of the underside of your cheekbone ledge, deepen the shadow by applying a narrow band of **dark 2** shadow cream **over** the original application of **dark 1** shadow cream.

This dual tone, if carefully applied and blended, will give the illusion of a real shadow that seems to deepen the hollow under the cheekbone. By deepening the cheekbone hollow and in combination with the **light** already applied on the top level of the cheekbone ledge (along with other techniques you will learn later in this book), you will create the illusion of a higher, rounded, sculpted cheekbone that will continue the direction of the brow line as a subtle frame encircling and spotlighting the eyes.

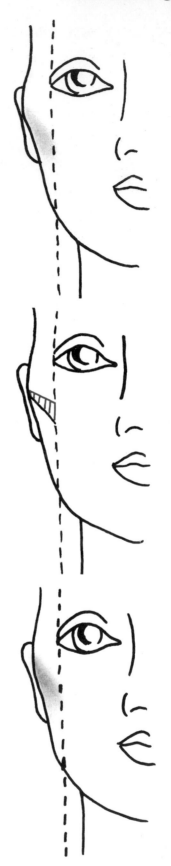

The third area to be shadowed is under the front tip of the chin and along the underneath edge of the jawbone. This placement of shadow tones—which deepens the natural shadow created by the jut of the chin and jawbone by seeming to project the face away from the neck and giving the face more importance—is not only for those with a slight fleshiness or a double chin but even for those with a firm, young jaw line which may be enhanced with a proper application of shadow creams.

Procedure

1. Again, two tones do the trick. First, using the point just underneath the edge of the jawbone as a guide for your finger movement, start at the base of the ear and sketch a line of **dark 1** toward the under edge of the tip of the chin. Then draw the same line on the other side and connect the points under the frontal tip of the chin.

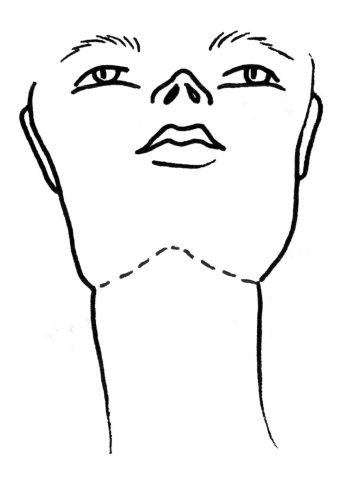

2. Connect the points from ear to ear along the horizontal line where the neck meets the chin so that when completed you have sketched the outline of a large triangle.

3. **Touch and press,** and lightly stroke downward to blend the shadow cream into the neck coloring. No line of demarcation should show at any of the edges of the triangle. Be careful not to move the shadow cream up onto the jawbone—which would defeat the purpose of enhancing the shadow that occurs naturally; rather, keep the **dark 1** shadow cream **underneath** the bottom side of the ledge created by the jawbone and chin.

4. **Dark 2** shadow cream may be applied in the very center of the triangle —particularly if one has a double chin or loose flesh in that area—to deepen the shadow and minimize the appearance of excess flesh.

The fourth area where shadow creams may be applied is the eye and temple area, but I'll discuss this in a subsequent chapter about shaping, strengthening visual impact, and enlarging the appearance of the eyes.

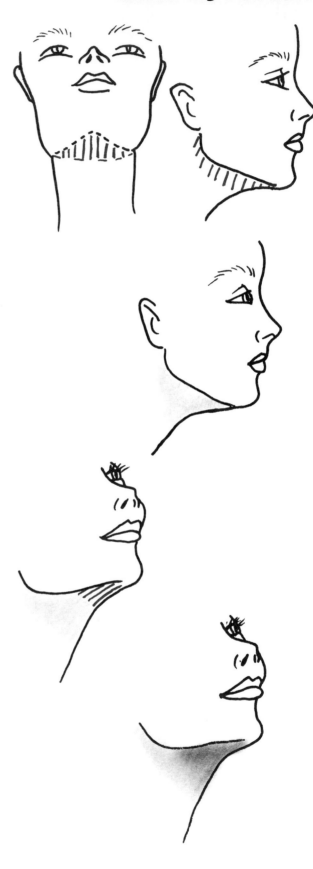

Color Glow

Color is a vital element in brightening and contouring a SCULPTURE-POR-TRAIT. Whereas **light** seems to project bones and **dark** seems to recede them, colors in the red range do something else. Not only does color give accent to the area where it is placed but it also seems to round out, give curve and softness to the skin and bones where it is applied. I call this combination of effects **color glow.**

A fluid in a bottle or soft cream paste in a small pot which is a vivid, hot red (somewhere between the color of blood and Chinese lacquer) is my favorite medium for giving accent and the illusion of vitality to a face.

Bright, strong cosmetic color in a container is almost never so intense when blended into the skin, so don't be timid when selecting reds.

To help understand why and how to use color, observe the faces of babies and healthy young people after exercise. One can almost see the flow of rich warm blood under the surface of the skin. A glow of color appears on the cheeks, perhaps on the sides of the neck, the tip of the chin, sometimes on the top of the forehead near the temples, and across the bridge of the nose. Obviously, this pattern is a natural guide for placement of cosmetic color to simulate the glow of health, the flush of youth.

Again, you use the vertical dotted line running perpendicular to the outside corner of the eye as a guide for exact placement of **color glow** on the side **ledge** of the cheekbone. Already you have placed and blended **light** on the top of the cheekbone and **dark** underneath the bottom of the cheekbone ledge. Now, the area of the cheekbone between the **light** and the **dark**—the **side** of the ledge—is the place for **color glow.**

Procedure

1. Starting on the front of the cheekbone at the imaginary vertical dotted guideline and moving backward to the hairline, use a fingertip to dot three small circles of **color glow.**

2. Use the **touch and press** method to blend the **color glow.** There should be no line of demarcation or of separation between the three levels of contouring—**light, dark,** and **color glow.** The blending must be so perfect that someone observing the finished work will have no awareness of the specific areas of placement. The illusion of a softly rounded, prominent cheekbone should be all that is apparent to the beholder.

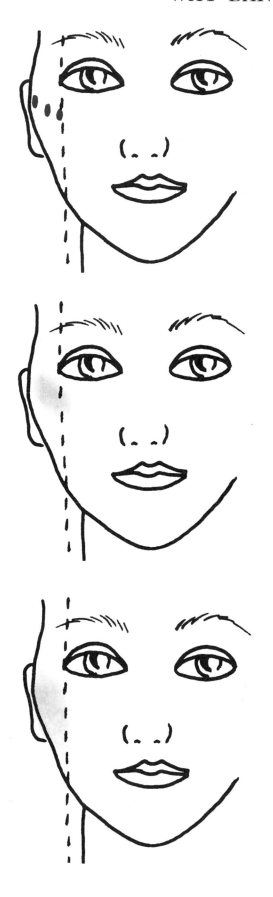

3. A tiny dot of **color glow** very carefully blended in the following places can help to create the appearance of a sunny, healthy flush of youth:

—the tip of the chin

—over the peak of each brow near the temples

—along the sides of the neck beneath the ear lobes

—on the high frontal bridge of the nose (this is very tricky and should be avoided by all but the unquestionably expert)

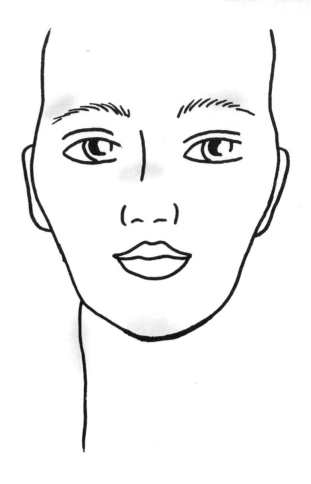

One must be very cautious when applying cosmetics to the neck area. If not thinned and blended and lightly applied, cosmetics on the neck not only can appear to be unclean and a bit ridiculous but can also soil clothes. Only after you have perfected the techniques of applying and blending **color glow** to the cheekbones should you attempt it on other areas of the face and neck. Again, like shaping the nose with shadow creams, many of the **color glow** frills of your SCULPTURE-PORTRAIT should be reserved for evening use or for times when you are being photographed professionally.

Powder

Face powder, properly chosen and carefully applied, can act as a filter does in photography. Powder seems to minimize imperfections and blend harsh edges and give an overall soft, velvety-appearing finish to a SCULPTURE-PORTRAIT. The key phrases here are "properly chosen" and "carefully applied."

Choose a baby talcum or finely milled talcum that is white in appearance but when applied to the skin is actually transparent. It should add **no color** to the face and, more important, should not change the colors of other cosmetics already on the skin.

A very soft "blush-on" brush or powder brush with washable bristles is the best tool for applying powder to the face. You should have two or three brushes so that you can wash the brush after each use and allow drying time before its next use. (A hair dryer does the trick in a pinch.) A second brush of the same type should be clean and available for touch-ups during the day or evening, and still a third brush should be ready for use at your worktable.

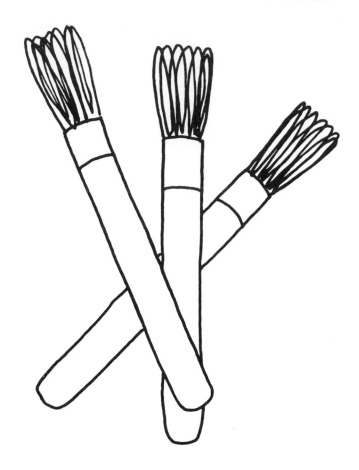

Did you ever consider the unsanitary condition of a powder puff used over and over throughout each day to blot up excess oil over a period of several months? After trying clean brushes, can you ever again feel comfortable using a powder puff or sponge on your face more than once? And puffs generally hold too much powder for effective application. Cotton balls or pads, on the other hand, have the advantage of one-time use but the annoying disadvantage of leaving fine threads or fuzz on the face.

The ideal powder container is a salt shaker with a top that can be closed

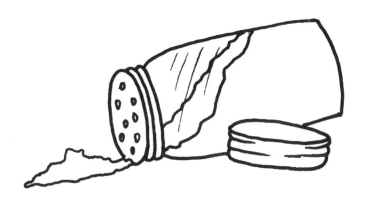

to prevent the powder from spilling through the holes when not in use. Perhaps you can find a small one to take with you for touch-ups.

Procedure

1. Shake a small amount of powder into the palm of your left hand (vice versa if you are left-handed).

2. With the soft powder brush, take up some of the powder from your palm and rather vigorously shake or flick excess powder from the brush. When no powder falls from the brush as you shake it, the excess powder has been removed.

3. Very delicately stroke the brush across the face as if you were touching a newborn baby. You should think that you are very lightly **buffing** the skin surface. Start under the eyes, across the cheekbones, the forehead, eyelids, nose, and then over the rest of the lower face, chin, and neck.

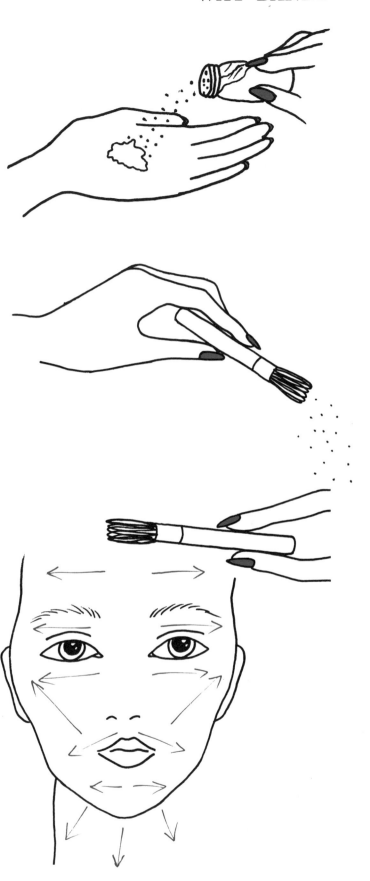

43

You may have to take up more powder on the brush once or twice during
the application; however, at no time
should you fail to shake the excess
powder from the brush, or you will
apply too much powder and spoil all
the effort you have put into your
SCULPTURE-PORTRAIT.

This method of applying powder
achieves the purpose of setting and
slightly dulling the shine of the cream
and fluid products on the skin. Using
transparent baby talcum in the way
I have described removes the **shine**
but leaves the **sheen.** There is no flat,
dry powdered look; the skin glows
with a kind of radiance—very attractive and very natural in appearance.

Later, in another lesson, you will have
instructions for doing a complete
SCULPTURE-PORTRAIT using only
powder products and employing many
of the techniques you have already
learned.

Eyes

Everyone seems to want large, bright, beautifully shaped eyes. And many people have them—what a blessing! Often a face with no other marks of beauty is thought to be beautiful because of extraordinary eyes. All other parts of the face we have talked about involve skin and bones. But to enhance the eyes we must work with the skin and bones around the eyes.

It has been my experience that using eye color products such as blue and green shadows seems to **conquer** rather than enhance one's own eye color. The color pigment in the cosmetic product always seems to be more vulgar in intensity than the gentle tones mother nature blended in the iris of the eye. Consequently, I suggest that you use delicate, soft blends of tan, brown, grey and beige shadow creams to exaggerate and define the shape and size of the eyes, because these shades also work to intensify the natural coloration of your eyes. However, if you must use other colors of eye cosmetics, the **patterns of application** presented in this chapter will still apply for your eye design.

Remember way back in the eyebrow lesson when I discussed **framing** the eye? Then, later, I suggested the exaggeration of the cheekbone to continue the eyebrow curve as a frame to spotlight the eyes. Even the vertical lines of shadow cream on the sides of the nose complete the framing as they direct the viewer's eye back to the beginning of the eyebrow. Do you begin to **see** the framing of the eye—almost as if the eye is being spotlighted, given paramount importance?

Perhaps you have noticed that when dealing with individual bone structure to create a SCULPTURE-PORTRAIT, such questions as face **shapes** (that is, square face, round face, etc.) become irrelevant. Each face is totally individual and has its own beauty potential that is not based on any norm, such as an "oval" face shape.

The same individuality applies to the eyes. Do not be concerned about deepset, protruding, or any other type of eyes. My techniques for framing the eyes will simply give the illusion of enlarging and exaggerating the shape and vitality of the eyes.

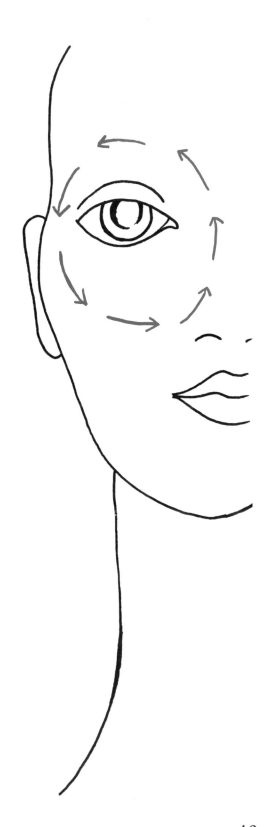

Procedure

1.   Cover the entire area from lashes to eyebrows with a very light application of **dark 1** shadow cream dotted on and then blended by **touching and pressing** with a fingertip.

2.   Cover the eyelid up to the crease (at the top of the eyeball) and just slightly up onto the edge of the orbital bone with **dark 2** shadow cream (applied right over the **dark 1**). The top edge of the area covered by **dark 2** shadow cream should conform in shape to the curve of the opened top eyelid line that was the guide in an earlier lesson for shaping the under curve of the eyebrow.

Both the shadow creams should come down to the top edge of the **light** triangle which you applied to the top ledge of the cheekbone. At this point where **light** and **dark** meet, blending must be so carefully done that one is not aware of where the **light** stops and the **dark** begins.

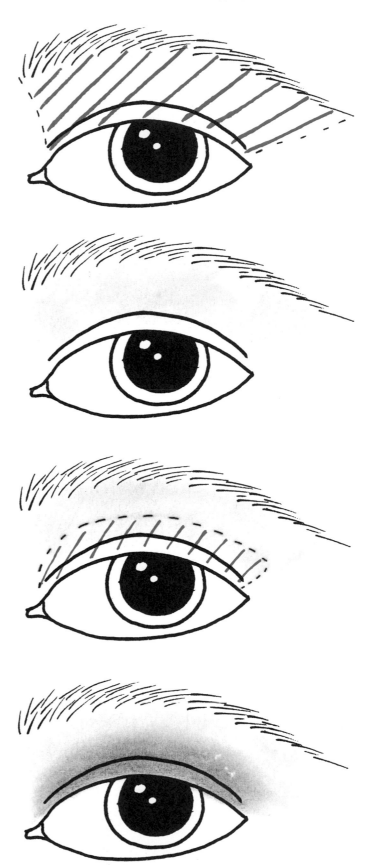

The shadow cream applications should begin not quite at the inside corner of the eye but slightly away (perhaps one-fourth inch) from the very inside corner at the point where eyelashes begin to grow.

3. Sketch a delicate line of charcoal-grey eyeliner among and **slightly** below the lower eyelashes and carry the line out just beyond the outside corner of the eye to meet the **dark** shadow creams you have applied above the eye. Carefully smudge/blend the charcoal pencil line with a fingertip or a cotton-tipped swab until it is imperceptible as a definite line and only serves to give the impression of thickening the lower eyelashes. Again, this smudged pencil line should begin where the lower eyelashes start growing, slightly away from the inside corner of the eye.

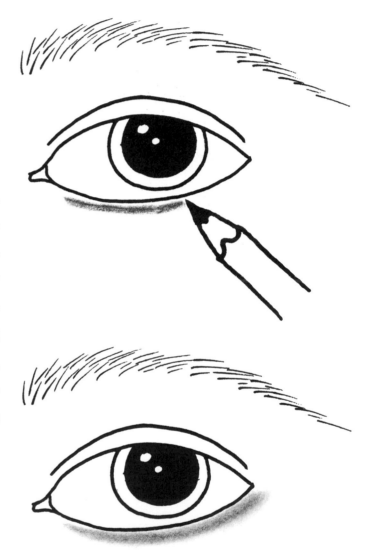

4. Place the index finger of the hand you do not work with on the top of one eyelid and gently lift the eyelid up and away so that the tiny rim of flesh just underneath the eyelashes is exposed to your mirror. With a black eye-liner pencil sketch a line along this rim inside your upper lashline (underneath the top eyelashes) from the inside corner (where the eyelashes begin to grow) to the outside corner of the eye.

The purpose is to define the shape of the eye without the eye liner showing. A touch of pencil liner may be applied **among** and very slightly **over**. the lashes to supplement density. Any liner above the lashes must be smudged with a fingertip or cotton-tipped swab to prevent a definite line.

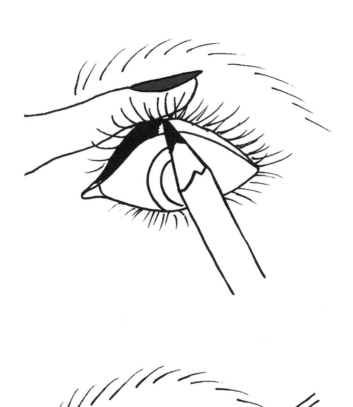

If you wear contact lenses it is imperative to keep the eye free of debris to avoid cloudy vision or discomfort. Therefore, you may wish to smudge the pencil liner only **among** and **over** the eyelashes rather than inside the upper lash line. However, many clients of mine who wear contact lenses have no problem after the initial few minutes necessary for the tear glands to water and "settle" the eye after the pencil liner is applied inside the upper lash line. If the pencil liner does not work for you, try a cake eye liner which requires a very fine eye-liner brush for application; use sterile eye drops rather than water as a wetting solution for the eye liner.

There is no need to adjust cosmetic application if you wear eyeglasses. Actually, the magnification of eyeglasses very often intensifies the effect of cosmetics applied around the eyes, so it is certainly not usually necessary to add more eye cosmetics (as we have often been advised editorially). Rather, proceed with your SCULPTURE-PORTRAIT as if you do not wear eyeglasses. Haven't you noticed that many eyeglass wearers use their glasses as an accessory with which they emphasize gestures in conversation? Often, in fact, the eye glasses seem to be off as much as they are on.

5.   Use an eyelash curler to curve the top eyelashes up and out, to open the eye like rays of the sun. Here is a technique that facilitates the job. Rather than clamping the curler and holding it closed on the eyelashes for a minute or more as many people tend to do, place the curler at the base of the lashes and make several firm, insistent squeezes. Relax pressure between squeezes but don't change the position of the curler.

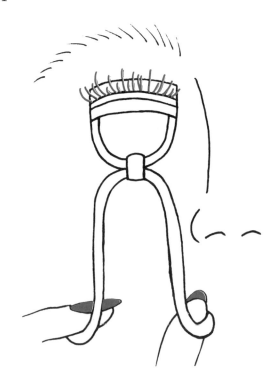

6. Using black mascara with a brush wand, darken each eyelash from the base to the tip, top and bottom. If you rest your little finger against your chin to steady your support and move the tip of the brush wand **horizontally** (rather than sweeping it upward), you may find it easier to coat each eyelash more evenly without getting mascara on the skin around the eyes.

If you do make a mistake, immediately remove the spot of mascara from the skin with a cotton-tipped swab. After mascara is applied, brush through the lashes in the direction they grow (upward and outward) with a mascara brush (or child's toothbrush) to separate the lashes and prevent that gloppy, stuck-together, spiky look. Remember, you are using mascara to color each eyelash darker—not to create new lashes. And not to curl the eyelashes—the eyelash curler has already achieved that.

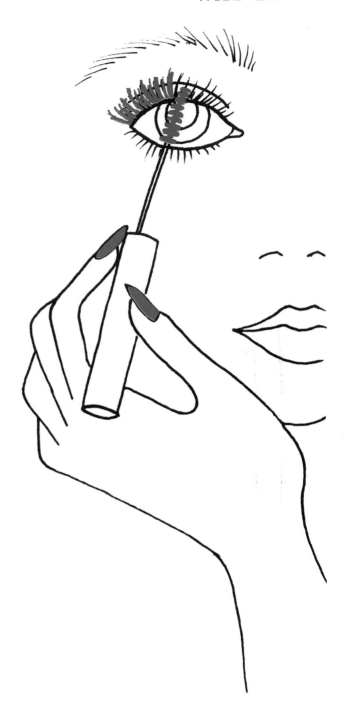

51

7. At this point, apply pencil color to the eyebrow and groom the hairs upward with a brow brush as described in the eyebrow lesson.

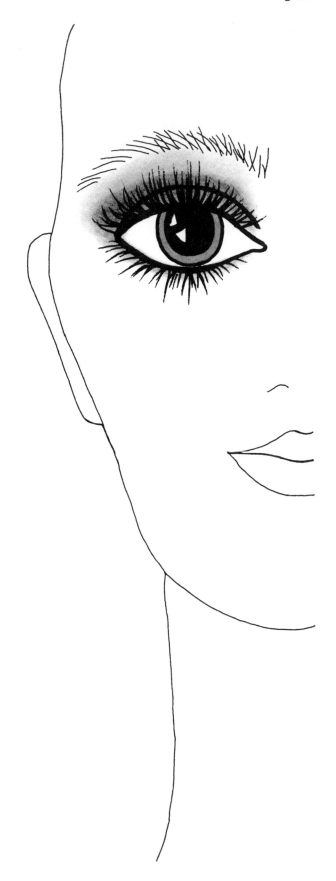

Artificial Eyelashes

You should only consider artificial lashes for street wear if you have practically no lashes and need to use artificial ones. Even then, they should only be applied in tiny individual clumps or sections to fill in and/or supplement sparse eyelash growth.

Although much dexterity is required for successful application of these small pieces of artificial eyelashes, you'll be rewarded with the splendor of full, thick eyelashes, almost indistinguishable from the real thing, when you perfect the technique—but **only** if you follow these directions carefully. Two key elements for success are that the artificial lashes must be made of human hair in a blend of brown and black and that you must hold neatness and precision paramount during the application procedure.

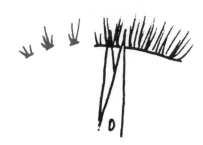

Procedure

1. Using small straight-tipped scissors, snip through the base of a standard strip of eyelashes, at regular intervals, to get several small "sections" of lashes, three or four hairs to a section and each still attached to a tiny piece of base strip.

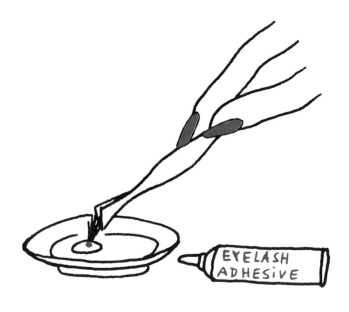

2. Now put a large drop of eyelash adhesive on a small plate near the mirror on your worktable. Using tweezers to grip the hair tips of one of the shortest-haired sections (cut from the short-haired inside corner of the standard eyelash strip), touch the base strip of the section to the eyelash adhesive; shake it in the air for a moment to set the adhesive; then attach the tiny section by its base strip to the skin of the eyelid, nestling it among the real eyelashes near the inside corner of the eye where the lashes start growing.

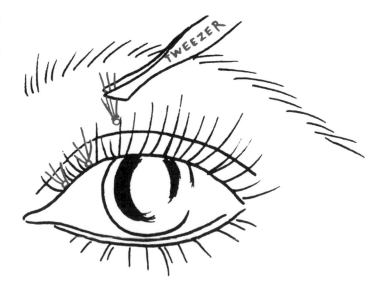

Continue placing tiny, individual sections at regular intervals along the eyelash line. Always be sure to place shorter-haired sections where shorter eyelashes really grow and longer-haired sections where longer eyelashes grow (longer lashes grow at the center of the eye and along the outer half of the eyelid). These artificial, individually applied sections of eyelashes should be applied after the real eyelashes have been curled but before mascara is applied. It may be necessary to trim any exceptionally long artificial hairs by snipping very cautiously with the tiny scissors.

Applying mascara will blend (and help to secure) the artificial lashes with the real lashes so the fake ones are even more undetectable.

To remove the artificial lashes, simply pull them gently with the fingertips or tweezers, being cautious not to pull out any of the precious real eyelashes. A bit of oil will help to loosen the eyelash adhesive. Individually applied artificial eyelashes should be cut and applied fresh each day. Using them a second time is both difficult and unclean because of the adhesive and mascara left from the first wearing.

Lips

The rosy, moist softness of a baby's lips should be the guide for emphasizing the mouth of your SCULPTURE-PORTRAIT. That is the ideal. And if your mouth is full, soft, and definite in shape and color, just mix a tiny drop of red transparent fluid or **color glow** with clear lip gloss and apply it to your mouth with a lip brush. However, most mouths are not so lucky—and they need more help.

Fashion changes and new lip colors are favored from time to time, but the most appealing mouths are time and again those that look "kissable." We all seem to thrive on change, exaggeration, adornment, and I am all for it! But don't you think it is smart to know how to make a beautiful, easy, soft, pretty mouth when you're in the mood to be kissed? For your beautiful new mouth design, just look on the next page and get to work...

Remember finding the center of those horizontal lines representing your nostrils which you used as guides for shaping the nose with shadow creams? Now that same central point of each nostril will be your starting-point guide for shaping a beautiful mouth.

Procedure

1. Using a very sharp auburn or light reddish-brown pencil, draw two dots at the points just at the edge of the upper lip and straight down from the exact center of each nostril.

Continue down across the lips and draw two more dots at the edge of the bottom lip.

2. Connect the dots at the edges of the upper and lower lips with two exactly straight vertical lines.

Draw arbitrarily straight lines ignoring the valleys and the mountains of the mouth contour—again, pretend you are drawing on a flat surface.

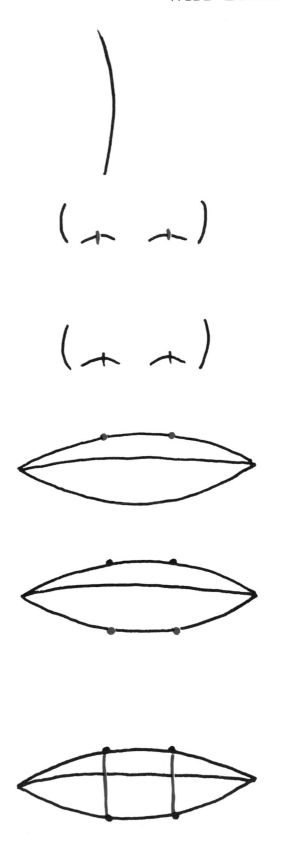

3. Now draw a shorter vertical line only on the top lip exactly in the center of the two other vertical lines.

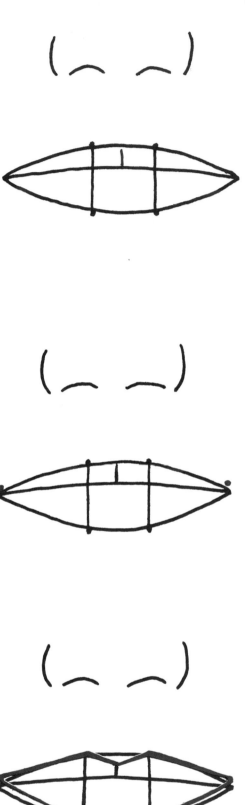

4. Place a dot with the auburn pencil at each outside corner of the mouth but ever so slightly above the real exact corner.

These dots must be placed so fractionally above the outside corners of the mouth that they are almost imperceptible. But this very slight raising of the mouth corners will tend to give you a pleasant expression even when the mouth is in repose.

5. Now all you must do is connect the dots with **straight** lines using the auburn pencil.

Sounds easy, doesn't it? Well, it will be with practice, but the first few times you may be awkward. Drawing straight lines on a flat surface is one thing; drawing straight lines on a curved surface is another.

Try it on a friend's mouth to help gain dexterity and understanding of this remarkable technique. Eventually, you will place the dots without drawing the guidelines across the lips from top to bottom; then, finally you will **know** your new mouth shape so completely that you will no longer need the dots as a guide.

Obviously, the guidelines should become a very delicate suggestion of shape as you improve and you should save your new mouth for public approval until you have mastered this trick.

6. Now for coloring the lips. At the base of an index finger (the one that you do not work with) place three tiny dabs of the following colors:

—**dark 1** shadow cream
—red transparent fluid or red cream rouge (**color glow**)
—clear lip gloss

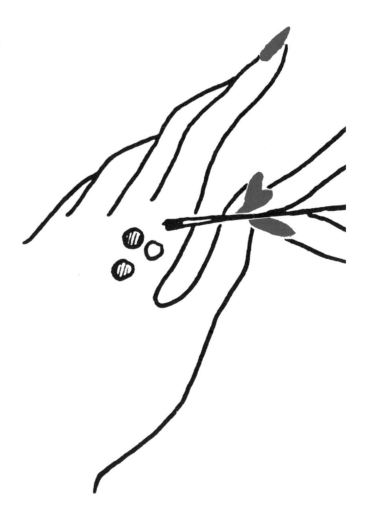

7. Using a square-tipped lip brush, mix these three colors to form one new color, which will be a soft, neutral, warm rose-beige of smooth texture and moist consistency.

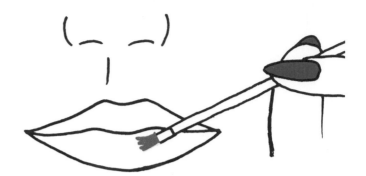

8. With the lip brush apply this lip color you have mixed to the entire mouth shape covering the auburn pencil lines and blending them with the lip color so that the lip outline is not apparent. Finally, apply a small amount of clear lip gloss to the lower lip for a moist, appealing fullness and sheen.

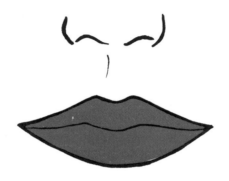

After-Five Face

Now that you have begun to learn how to bring your facial skin and bones to what I consider to be "peak" daytime beauty, you may be wondering about what to do when you go out in different lighting in the evening.

Already I have suggested that certain of the shading techniques using **dark 1** and **dark 2** are best left for professional photography sessions or for very dimly lighted restaurants and rooms.

For my eye there is no such thing as "evening cosmetics." All one really needs to do is to use slightly more intense applications of the cosmetic techniques you have learned for your daylight SCULPTURE-PORTRAIT.

That is—more **color glow,** more darkness in shaping the eyes, more **light** on the top ridge of the cheekbone ledge, perhaps more red in the lip color mixture, and certainly more mascara and lip gloss.

So you see that one may go from work to dinner without changing the face entirely by starting over to build a new SCULPTURE-PORTRAIT. You need only to intensify for evening lighting. After all, you have very carefully selected the colors that enhance your beauty; and you have very exactingly plotted your sculptural design to bring your face to optimum symmetry. So, as the light falls you will simply turn up the color volume . . . and have a beautiful evening.

Powder Portrait

It is possible to create a SCULP-TURE-PORTRAIT using only powders of various colors. The softness, ease of blending, and lack of oil content which are the attractive characteristics of powder products can be very satisfying and effective for those who dislike the feel of liquids and creams on the skin.

Some disadvantages of powders as opposed to liquids are the difficulty of specific placement; the effect on some skins of dryness and fine wrinkles that powder, improperly applied to skin that has not been properly pre-pared, may cause; and the "patchiness" of coloration caused by the "drag" of colored powders over dry skin areas.

And yet, despite these disadvantages, if you have mastered the lessons for creating a SCULPTURE-PORTRAIT using liquids and creams, you can also learn to work effectively with powders.

The face reflects a lovely soft translucent effect when colored powders are properly mixed and applied to enhance the facial skin and bones.

You will need the following equipment in addition to that already on your worktable (see, I promised you *more*):

—a translucent no-color baby talcum
—a yellow-beige loose powder in a shade as close as possible to your naked skin color
—a warm-toned red loose powder
—a pure-white loose powder
—a warm-toned bronze loose powder
—a cool-toned dark earth-brown loose powder
—a very light-textured non-oily protective skin lotion
—a spray of distilled or pure mineral water

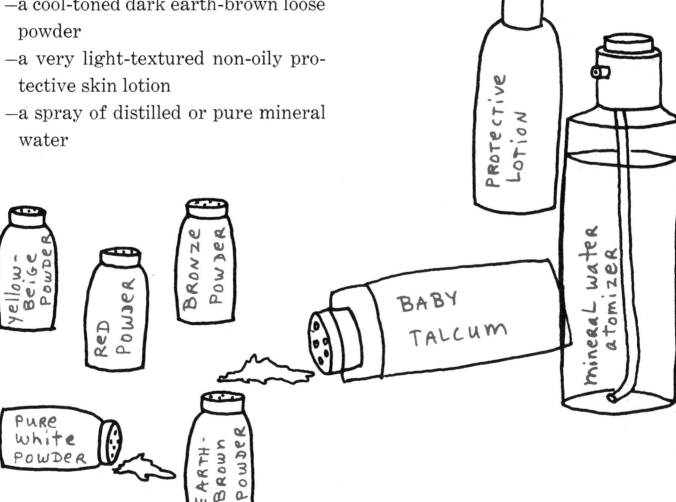

You may have to make your own loose powders by grinding pressed-powder blush-ons and pressed-powder eye-shadows with a mortar and pestle or, in a pinch, with a kitchen knife handle in a glass bowl. An artist's palette knife may also be useful for mixing and blending powders.

You will need at least two soft powder brushes for each color of powder.

As suggested in the earlier powder lesson, you may use salt shakers as loose powder containers.

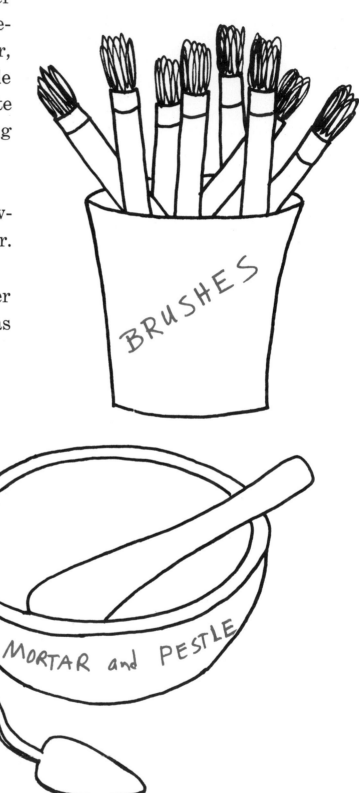

BRUSHES

ARTIST PALETTE KNIFE

MORTAR and PESTLE

Procedure

1.   Apply protective skin lotion to the surface of the entire face and neck and wait a few minutes for absorption.

2.   Mist the face with distilled or mineral water and blot delicately with a soft cloth to remove all traces of lubrication and water.

3.   In a small jar, mix the following powders to form one new powder color:

—one-half teaspoon red loose powder
—one-quarter teaspoon bronze loose powder
—three tablespoons baby talcum
—three teaspoons yellow-beige loose powder

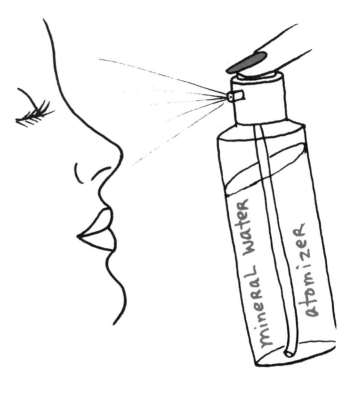

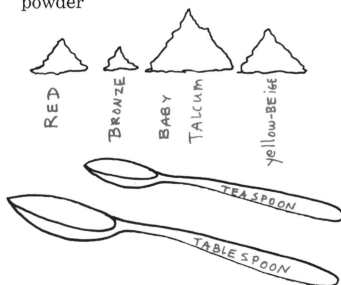

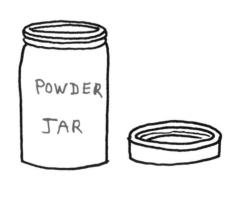

Shake the closed jar vigorously for a minute or two until all the powder colors have mixed to form one new glowing, warm-toned, flesh-tinted loose powder. It may be necessary to grind this mixture with mortar and pestle to achieve a really fine blend. You will, of course, wish to mix these powder formulas before you begin your powder SCULPTURE-POR-TRAIT, but I list them here in the **procedure** for the sake of continuity.

4. With a soft powder brush, **buff** onto the entire face a very light application of translucent no-color baby talcum. Always use the technique (described in the powder lesson) of shaking excess powder from the brush before touching it to the skin. This application of talcum acts as a base for all the other powder products. It is much easier to apply and blend colored powders on this base of talcum than onto naked skin.

5. Using another brush, buff onto the skin a thin, thin application of the loose powder color you mixed in Step 3 of this procedure.

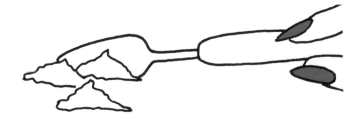

6.   Mix in equal parts (one teaspoon each) baby talcum, yellow-beige powder, and the pure-white powder and apply with a small soft brush in all those areas where you learned to apply **light** to give the illusion of "lifting forward" unattractive valleys of the facial landscape.

7.   Using the bronze loose powder as **dark 1** and the earth-brown loose powder as **dark 2,** shape the mountains of the face structure just as you learned to do in the **dark** lesson and in the **eyes** lesson.

8.   Mix equal parts of bronze and yellow-beige powders, and add a pinch of earth-brown powder. Using a tiny, stiff flat-edged brush, feather-stroke the resulting new color of powder to shape the eyebrows.

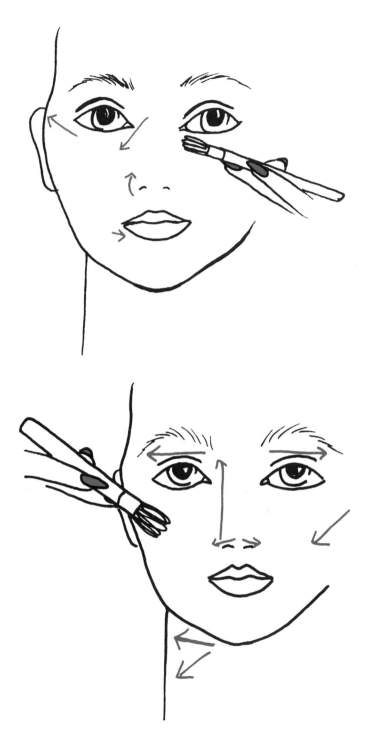

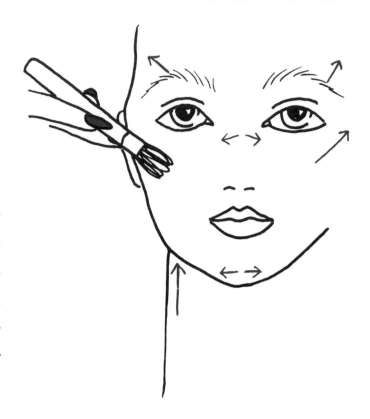

9. Mix equal parts of red powder and yellow-beige powder, and apply to the face with a soft brush in the same places as you learned to do in the **color glow** lesson.

10. For a misty blending, give a final buff over the entire face with baby talcum. Then use (as you have already learned to do) the black eyeliner pencil, black mascara, eyelash curler, and cream lip colors to complete your POWDER SCULPTURE-PORTRAIT.

When you have learned these powder techniques well, you may enjoy doing a very beautiful—but less precise—creation in just a few minutes. However, keep in mind the disadvantages of using only powders, and practice until you are certain of your skill before showing your new POWDER SCULPTURE-PORTRAIT to the world.

Pressed powders, such as blush-ons and eyeshadows, become loose powders when taken up on a brush before applying them to the face. However, I prefer the less heavy, less dense quality of finely milled loose powders shaken from a container in the hand. The loose powder seems to be lighter, fluffier, and sheerer on the skin.

It has been my experience that desirable shades of pressed powders that work properly to define complexion colorations and to shape facial planes are difficult to find. Therefore, until such pressed powder products are commercially available, it is preferable to grind and mix one's own loose powders.

Skin

We live in an age when an attractive appearance seems to be important and we use cosmetics because they help us not only to look better but to feel better.

Many of us are aware that most commercial cosmetics contain ingredients that may be abusive to the balance of nature as related to the health of our skin. But we also realize that truly natural cosmetics either do not exist or, if they do exist, are economically unfeasible and not readily available to the general public.

Therefore, until the time comes when we can "have our cake and eat it too," the information in this chapter will help you to cleanse and treat your skin naturally but still allow you to use cosmetics as suggested in this book.

The less one does to normal, healthy skin the better it will look. The key words here are "normal, healthy." And you know if you have it or if you don't.

If one learns as a child the balance of nature in effective nutrition, the results are clearly manifest as radiant physical health. Unfortunately, most standard medical and educational information does not express effective nutritional practices, so most of us do not have the advantage of a lifelong cooperation with the natural laws of nutrition. Some who search are rewarded with knowledge that leads to health, both internally and externally.

Cooperation with nature (even in the most sophisticated laboratory techniques) is the only basis for really effective beauty treatments.

Treatment of normal, healthy skin consists simply of splashing the face once or twice a day with first warm and then cool water. However, apply a commercial (or even a natural) cosmetic to the skin and it can no longer be classified as "normal, healthy." Anything you put into or onto your body has chemical qualities that will affect you. Have you ever read the ingredients on a cosmetic container? Do you know what you are putting on your skin? If so, do you begin to understand how cooperation with nature when cleaning and treating your skin is the only way to reclaim some balance after you have chemically abused the skin by using cosmetics?

I have found through research and experience over the years that the following program of cleaning and protecting the skin with natural products is the safest and most effective. As you apply the knowledge gained from the nutrition chapter your skin will respond even more dramatically to the following procedures.

Facial Skin

Evening —

1. If you are wearing cosmetics, clean the skin with a thin natural oil (unrefined, cold-processed avocado oil or cold-pressed olive oil are effective). After applying and lightly massaging with the fingertips, remove the oil and cosmetics with damp cotton pads from which you have squeezed excess moisture. You may have to repeat this cleansing procedure to remove all cosmetics.

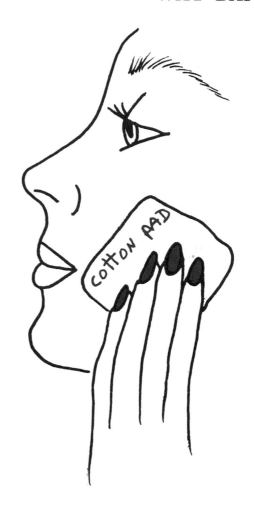

2. Using your fingertips, delicately apply 1 tablespoon of plain, natural yogurt to the entire face and neck and massage lightly before rinsing it away with warm water.

3. Moisten with water 1 teaspoon of yellow corn meal and **gently** scrub the entire face to loosen debris from the surface of pores and to remove dead skin cell accumulation.

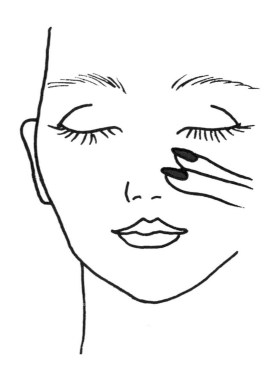

4. In a small bowl, mix ½ egg yolk (**not** egg white), ½ teaspoon honey, and 1 teaspoon plain yogurt—you may add a dash of cornstarch to thicken this mixture. Apply to the entire face and neck with the fingertips as a beauty mask. Be sure to apply as close to the eyes as possible—even the top lids. Leave the mask on for 15 minutes or longer. Then rinse off with warm water. When the mask is completely removed, rinse your face once more with a basin of warm water to which you have added 2 tablespoons of apple cider vinegar.

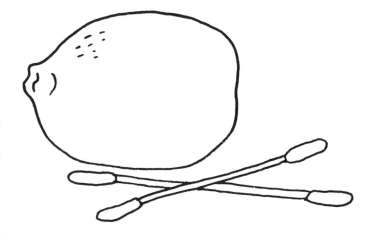

5. With a cotton-tipped swab, apply fresh lemon juice to any pimples or skin eruptions.

6. Do not apply cream to the entire face when you go to bed. However, at changes of seasons or if you seem to be particularly dry around the eyes, mouth, or neck when you go to another climate, you may apply a bit of thin avocado oil or a pure, natural lubricating cream or fluid.

Dr. Paavo O. Airola, in his book *How to Get Well*, gives the following formula for a natural skin treatment cream:

2 tablespoons sesame oil
1 tablespoon olive oil
2 tablespoons avocado oil
2 tablespoons almond oil
2,000 I.U. Vitamin E, mixed tocopherols
100,000 USP units Vitamin A

Pour the ingredients into a small bottle or jar. Close tightly and shake well. Keep refrigerated.

Morning —

1. Mist the face with noncarbonated mineral water. (A plant mister or an empty perfume atomizer is useful.)

2. After the mineral water dries, apply fresh lemon juice with a cotton-tipped swab to any pimples or skin eruptions and allow the juice to dry.

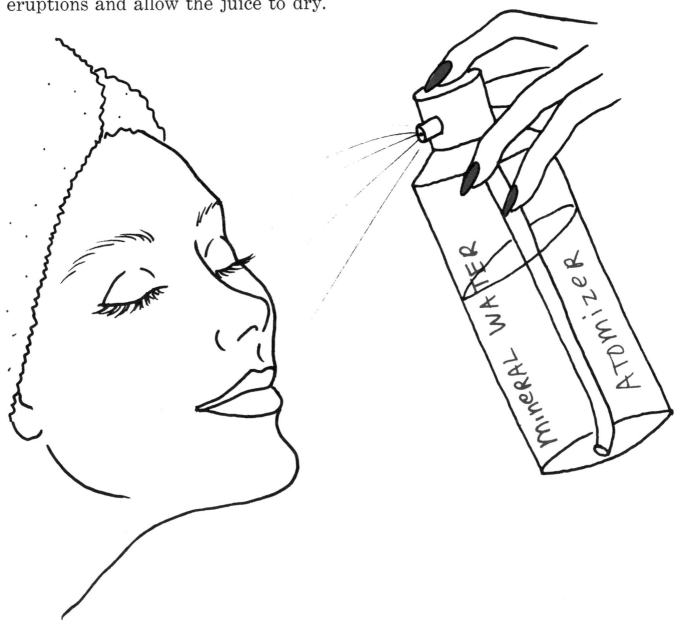

3. Apply a pure, natural protective skin lotion to any extremely dry areas of the face or neck. Wait 5 minutes for absorption; blot any excess with tissue and proceed with the **complexion prime coat.**

After using these skin treatments for a short while (especially if you are improving your body nutritionally at the same time) you will be rewarded with a skin to which you will apply cosmetics only for extra allure or enhancement. You will no longer require cosmetics for heavy coverage.

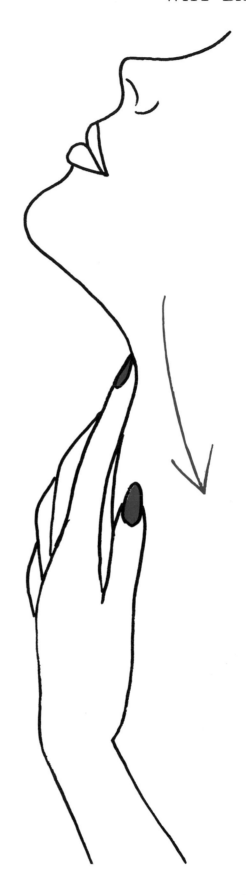

Body Skin

The skin has absorption capability and may receive moisturizing benefit from a daily tub bath. The skin may actually absorb cell-plumping water by osmosis. What is the quality of your bath water? Body fluids (blood, plasma, cell water) are chemically similar to sea water. Why not derive additional health benefits from your bath by adding a cup or more of sea salt to your bath water?

Baking soda is a natural neutralizer of body odors, so throw a few table-spoonfuls into your bath water. (There is some evidence that a combination of baking soda and sea salt in water may help to neutralize the effects of excess radiation to which we are exposed more and more in our environment.)

Apple cider vinegar added to your final rinse water helps restore protective acidity to the surface of the skin. A tablespoon or two is sufficient.

If you wish to bathe with a soap, your selection should be fortified with knowledge and experience. Very mild, low-detergent, non-alkaline, naturally scented cleansing bars are available in most stores that sell natural products. Even then, soap should be used only on the body areas that seem to accumulate odors—underarms, pelvic areas, feet. You may wish to keep a jar of yellow corn meal near your bathtub to smooth rough areas of the body such as feet, knees, and elbows, and to help remove dead skin cell accumulation.

Any body lotion used definitely must be derived from natural, pure ingredients. Can you imagine the insult to your body when you literally cover your skin with a lotion made entirely from artificial ingredients and synthetic emulsifiers and fragrances? How your body must struggle to restore balance as it absorbs the lotion!

Metallic and synthetic ingredients in commercial deodorants should be avoided—especially in glandular areas of the body, such as the underarms or the pelvic area, where deodorants are normally applied. And have you noticed that the more deodorant one uses, the more one seems to need?

Instead of using deodorants, you may be more satisfied with a cologne or toilet water made from natural (not synthetic, laboratory-derived) perfume essences.

Learn all that you can about the balance of nature, apply it on all levels of your existence, and reap the reward—an attractive, healthy body.

Sun

It is no news to anyone today that too much of our glorious sun's ultraviolet rays are damaging to human skin. And that damage is manifested externally as a dry, blotched, lined, leathery, prematurely aged complexion.

On the other hand, humans have not always worn clothes to walk this earth. Don't you think that a few minutes' exposure to the sun each day when weather permits must be harmonious with nature? Particularly if you can spend those few minutes in the sun each day completely without clothes?

We are all aware that exposure to sunlight is necessary for our body to produce its own Vitamin D. Perhaps the current vogue of encouraging us to fear the sun and its aging effects somewhat overstates the dangers.

The time to be on guard against sun damage is when you travel to a much sunnier, tropical or arid climate than your body is accustomed to. Unlimited exposure to stronger than usual (for you) ultraviolet rays from the sun requires unusual measures to protect the skin of your face and body from both temporary and long-range discomfort and damage.

Precautionary Measures

1. Limit sun exposure to a few minutes each day, certainly not more than 30 minutes. Use a kitchen timer or alarm clock to prevent sleeping for longer than you wish to sunbathe.

2. If you must be in the sun longer, cover your body with lightweight, light-colored but opaque loose clothing. Wear a ventilated hat (such as straw) that allows air to cool the head but still shades the face and neck to some degree.

3. In addition, the face, hands, and all other parts of the body exposed to the sun should be protected with a natural sun-screening lotion or cream. Know the ingredients before using the preparation. Usually some sun-screening products sold in health food stores list ingredients. Choose a product based on PABA (para-aminobenzoic acid), a natural sun-screening ingredient.

4. For moderate exposure to moderate sun, I have long used a homemade formula that seems to help prevent severe burning and to encourage a golden tone as the skin tans.

Recipe —

SUN EXPOSURE FLUID

Ingredients

1 cup noncarbonated mineral water
3 tea bags
3 tablespoons Aloe Vera Gel
Cheesecloth
¼ cup apple cider vinegar
1 glass atomizer bottle with plastic pump and lid

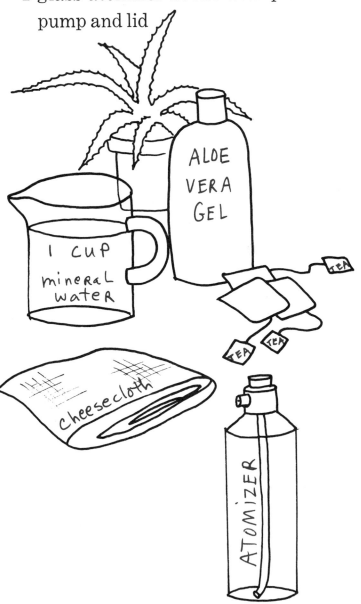

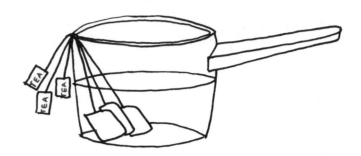

1. Heat 1 cup of noncarbonated mineral water to the boiling point and turn off heat.

2. Soak 3 tea bags in the heated water for 3 minutes; then remove the tea bags from the tea solution.

3. Strain 3 tablespoons of Aloe Vera Gel through a double layer of cheese-cloth. (Aloe Vera Gel may be obtained directly from the leaf of the aloe vera, or you may purchase bottled Aloe Vera Gel from health food stores.)

4. Pour the strained Aloe Vera Gel into a measuring cup containing ¼ cup of apple cider vinegar.

5. Add the Aloe/vinegar solution to the tea/water solution.

6. Strain the entire solution through two layers of cheesecloth into a large measuring cup with a pouring lip.

7. Pour the finished strained solution into a glass atomizer bottle and allow to cool to room temperature. The atomizer pump and lid to the bottle should be plastic rather than metal.

Mist this clear, amber-toned **sun exposure fluid** onto your face and body frequently as you take a daily short sunbath. After several days your skin will have a warm golden glow that will last well without serious damage from burning and drying.

The tannic acid from tea, the acidity of vinegar, and the protective, healing properties of Aloe Vera Gel assure you of some safety—but only if you are sensible and avoid overexposure.

A distinct disadvantage of the sun exposure fluid is the scent of vinegar, but the unpleasant smell seems to evaporate rather quickly. Perhaps you can solve the problem by suggesting that your sunbathing partners share your atomizer of sun exposure fluid.

Never, never use perfume or other fragrance products in the sun. Many fragrance ingredients may cause photosensitivity to the sun in some individuals which may result in areas of dark or light pigmentation on the face and/or body.

The second day after you make the sun exposure fluid it may appear to be cloudy. Do not be alarmed—it is still effective. But do make a new batch for the third day.

It is my opinion that oiling the skin in the sun is like basting meat in the oven. Oil seems to encourage burning rather than acting as protection.

It is when you come in from the sun that you should lubricate and moisturize the skin of your face and body to soften it and help prevent peeling and flaking.

Exercise

Exercising the muscles of the face, neck, and head in a controlled organized way improves blood circulation and thereby helps maintain the tone and contour of the facial skin and musculature. It will also "train" the muscles to control unattractive facial expressions. Sometimes the contours of the face can even be altered with concentrated and exaggerated attention to a particular area of the facial muscular structure, such as the muscles covering the cheekbones.

Just as an exercised body has a look of "fitness," so does an exercised face. If you walk five miles a day or jump rope ten minutes a day for a week, you will see and feel a difference in the tone of your body.

If you exercise your face daily for a week, you will experience a new awareness of contour and tone of the facial structure.

For several years I have experimented with many systems of facial exercise and have finally arrived at the following eight essential exercises for promoting and maintaining facial muscle tone and contour.

The movements require control and practice. To work, they must be done correctly.

Procedure

1. Secure hair back and away from the face.

2. Press hairsetting tape across the forehead to prevent wrinkling during the exercises. This step will be eliminated as your control progresses. At the beginning you may tape your forehead when you are alone around your house to develop awareness of how often you unconsciously wrinkle your forehead.

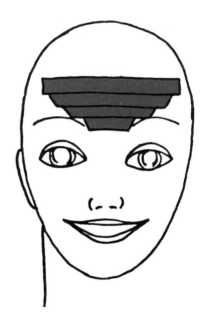

3. Lubricate the entire face and neck (except where you have taped the forehead, of course) with a rich, natural cream—perhaps Dr. Airola's formula (see page 73).

4. Repeat each exercise six times daily, six times a week for six weeks or longer until you feel you have trained the muscles and have control of your facial expressions. After that, three times a week tapering off to once a week should be enough for maintenance.

Exercises —

1. Start with mouth closed but do not clench teeth and do not tense lips. Using very tiny controlled movements, smile, moving the corners of your mouth toward the temples. The movements should not be choppy—think of them as a smoothly orchestrated progression. When you've gone as far as you can go, release the muscles in reverse, using the same ultracontrolled manner.

2. Begin with mouth slightly open, lips relaxed. A little at a time, and smoothly, wrinkle your nose upward very slowly as pictured. Release downward with definite, controlled movements.

3. A hard one to do with the proper amount of control, but try! Wrinkle your nose upward and hold tensely in that position while executing exercise number one. Concentrate! With control, release everything downward together. Don't let your face snap back fast.

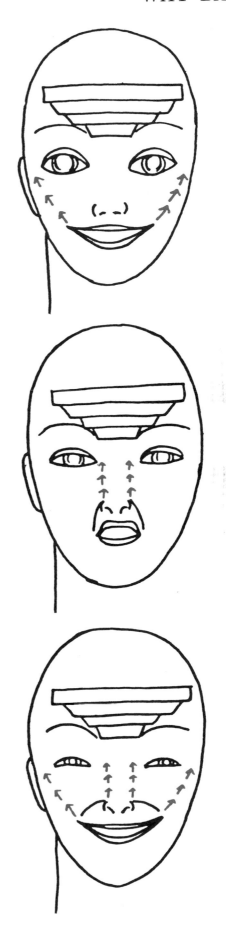

4.   This one takes a good deal of practice before you really feel what you are doing, so don't despair if you can't do it at all the first few times. It will come. Very slowly, as you focus your eyes upward, raise the lower lid inward and upward as illustrated by the arrows. Return to the starting position, remembering not to relax the muscles too quickly.

5.   To begin, drop your jaw and make an easy oval with your lips. Do not strain. Place your index finger on the chin for support. Execute exercise number four. The finger-on-chin maneuver adds resistance to the exercise and forces the muscles to work even more.

6.   Smooth extra cream on chin and neck. Bring jaw and lower teeth forward and up over upper teeth and lip. You must push the muscles in your chin up as high as you can. Do not move your lips at all as you push and relax. All the effort should come from the chin muscle.

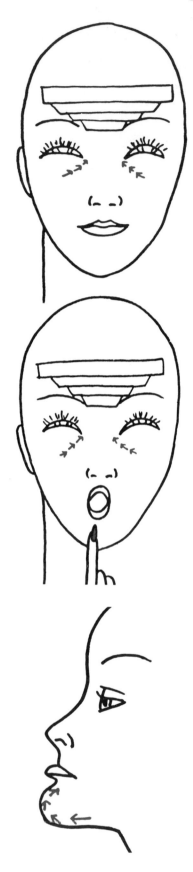

7. Place fists under chin as illustrated. Press up with your hands at the same time as you press down with your head, but do not allow either force to win. This one works on an isometric exercise principle.

8. Press index fingers firmly against eyebrows and attempt to lift the forehead muscles upward and back while using the finger pressure to prevent brows from lifting and forehead skin from crinkling. Do not use any other facial muscles. Relax everything except your fingers and your forehead. Eventually, you will be able to exercise forehead muscles without finger pressure on brows.

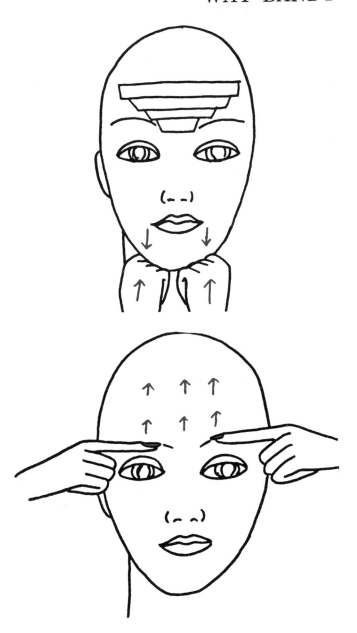

Nutrition

Consider your body as a delicate plant that only blooms under proper conditions of climate, nutrition, love, and that you are trying to grow a prize-winner without chemical fertilizers or poisonous sprays.

Health is nothing more than a life held in balance by natural conditions. It is that simple, but deceptively so. What, for example, is natural eating? It has taken me twenty years to begin to know. Each day I learn more. Perhaps you can benefit from my efforts and take a few shortcuts.

Modern civilization forces us into an unnatural way of living. We are so civilized and so removed from the basic laws of nature that we do not eat, drink, sleep, breathe or even clothe ourselves properly. Although our bodies adapt to changes in environment through the evolutionary process, the laws of the balance of nature are universal, permanent, unchanging; they must be obeyed, or the consequence will be sickness and disease. The human body does not sicken so long as it lives according to the laws of nature.

Even though these laws are simple, natural, obvious, we have moved so far from natural living that we must erase preconceived ideas and begin with a blank tablet, an open mind. We must each reeducate ourselves.

In these few pages only guidelines can be presented. You must use the reading list furnished at the end of this chapter to gain some understanding of why and how to live and eat according to the balance of nature.

Although we are extraordinary beings with unique physical characteristics and therefore require individual chemical and electromagnetic body analysis to arrive at our own formula for balanced living, here is a listing of nutritional guidelines that may get you started on the road back to natural eating patterns:

—Do not eat anything that has eyes to look back at you—except as a matter of survival. (Survival for some body and blood types may require animal protein.)

—Eat as many raw foods as possible (fruits, vegetables, nuts, seeds, sprouts).

—Do not mix fruits and vegetables at the same meal.

—Eat **eliminative** fruits and vegetables (dates, figs, celery, grapes, apricots, asparagus, etc.).

—Use whole grain rather than processed flour—avoid refined white sugar and white flour and everything made with them.

—Learn to prepare and combine foods to derive the most energy (fuel).

—Take **natural** (not laboratory-derived) vitamin and mineral supplements daily.

—Have your body chemistry analyzed by a naturopath (one who specializes in preventative and corrective medicine by treating with natural foods rather than with drugs).

—Do not eat or drink very hot or very cold foods or beverages.

—Develop several natural recipes for dishes you enjoy making quickly and easily.

—Use natural, raw, unheated, unfiltered, and unprocessed honey as a sweetener (rather than processed sugars or artificial sweeteners).

—Drink pure natural water (add ¼ teaspoon of sea salt to a quart of distilled water if you cannot get pure, uncontaminated, naturally mineralized spring water).

—Use cold-pressed vegetable oils.
—If you have a body that tolerates milk, use only certified raw milk rather than pasteurized milk.
—Eat only poison-free foods.
—Partake of food with a spirit of gratitude and love.

All fruits and vegetables may be treated in a special bath to destroy insecticides, germs, fungus, and metallics present in or on these foods and thereby to raise and restore the energy level of that food. If you would like the formula for this special food bath, refer to *The Electro-Magnetic Energy in Foods*, by Dr. Hazel Parcells.

If you adopt the above suggestions as a way of eating, the results will be so rewarding that you will want to know more. The following reading list will furnish you with what I believe to be the best available knowledge for natural living today:

The Electro-Magnetic Energy in Foods

by Dr. Hazel Parcells
Par-X-Cell School of Scientific Nutrition
1605 Coal Avenue, S.E.
Albuquerque, N.M. 87106

How to Get Well
by Dr. Paavo Airola
Health Plus Publishers
P.O. Box 22001
Phoenix, Ariz. 85028

The Best of Linda Clark
by Linda Clark
Keats Publishing, Inc.
36 Grove Street
Box 876
New Canaan, Conn. 06840

Yoga and Health
by Selvarajan Yesudian and Elisabeth Haich
Harper & Row Publishers, Inc.
10 East 53rd Street
New York, N.Y. 10022

Food Is Your Best Medicine
by Dr. Henry Bieler
Random House, Inc.
201 E. 50th Street
New York, N.Y. 10022

Mucusless Diet Healing System
by Arnold Ehret
Ehret Literature Publishing Co.
Beaumont, Calif. 92223

Diet for a Small Planet
by Frances Moore Lappe
Ballantine Books
201 E. 50th Street
New York, N.Y. 10022

Back to Eden
by Jethro Kloss
Lifeline Books
P.O. Box 1552
Riverside, Calif. 92502

You Are Extraordinary
by Roger J. Williams
Pyramid Publications
919 Third Avenue
New York, N.Y. 10022

Health for the Millions
by Herbert M. Shelton
Natural Hygiene Press, Inc.
205 West Wacker
Chicago, Ill. 60606

Sugar Blues
by William Dufty
Warner Books, Inc.
75 Rockefeller Plaza
New York, N.Y. 10019

Stalking the Wild Pendulum
by Itzhak Bentov
E. P. Dutton & Co., Inc.
201 Park Avenue South
New York, N.Y. 10003

The following pages are for your personal notes about designing *your* face. As you experiment with the techniques I've outlined in this book, mark down your findings. With experience, you'll learn what combination of cosmetics is exactly right for you.

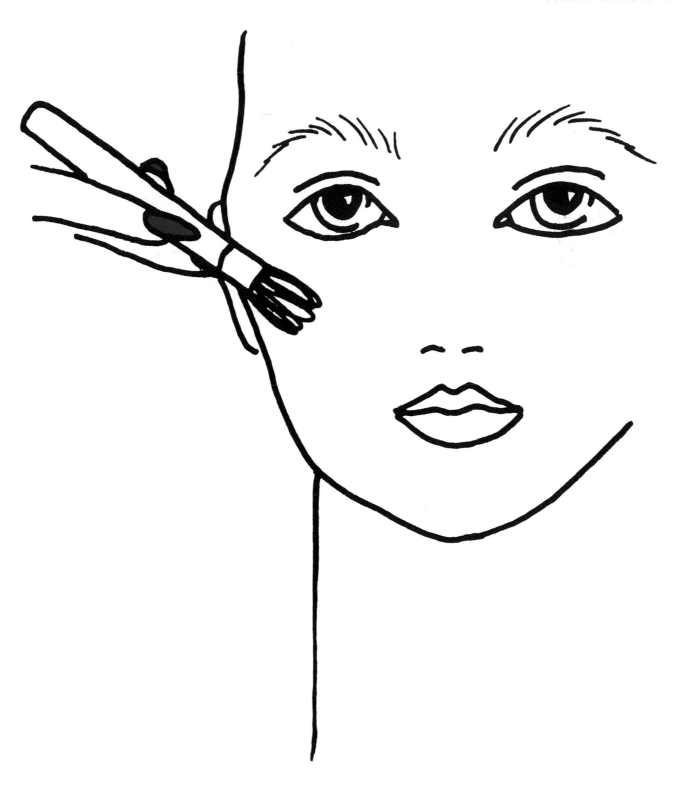

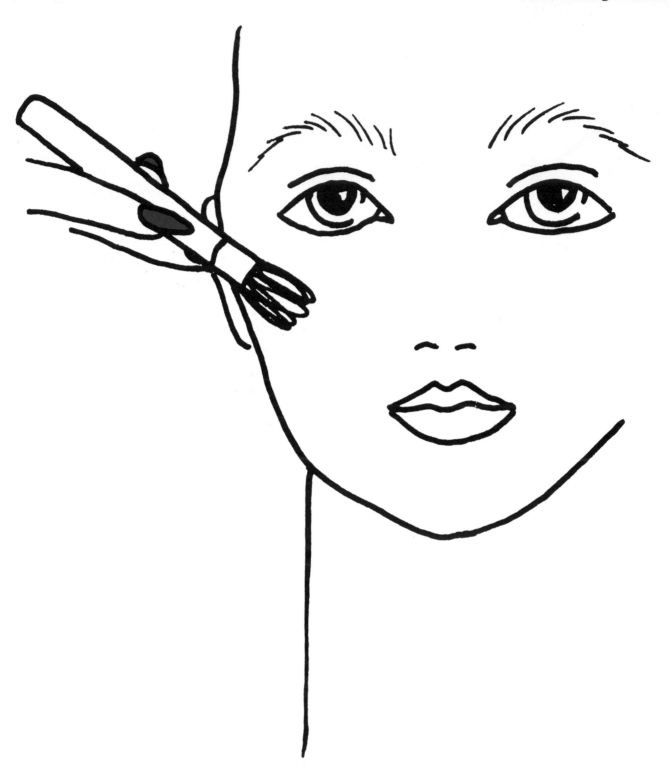

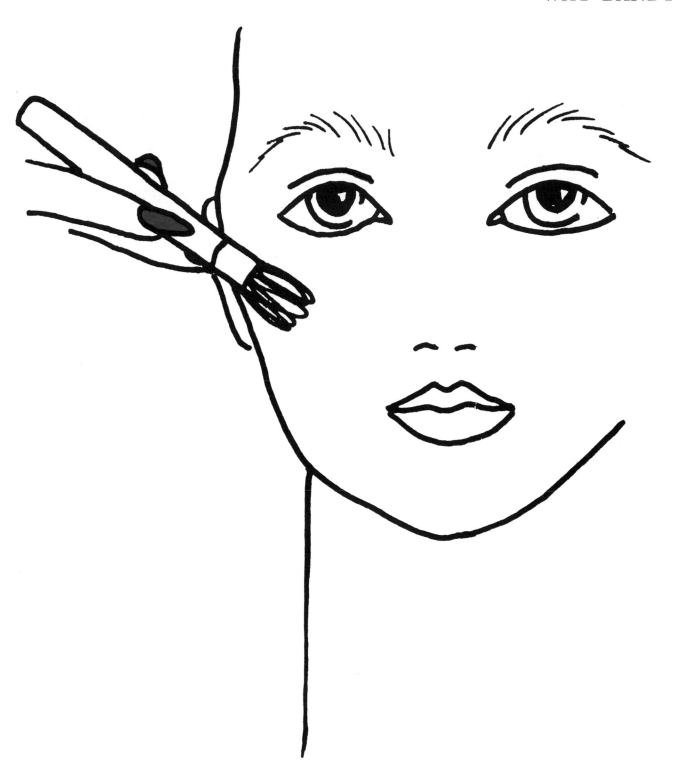

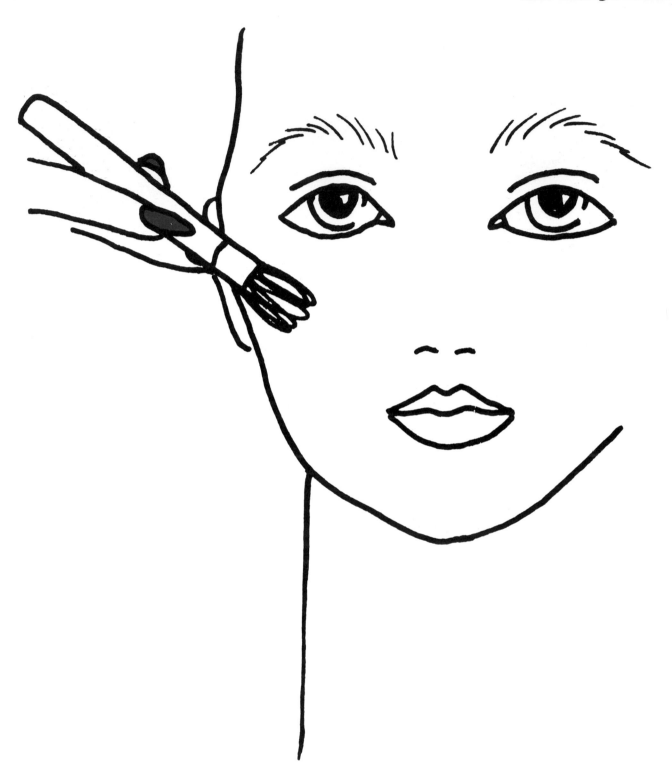

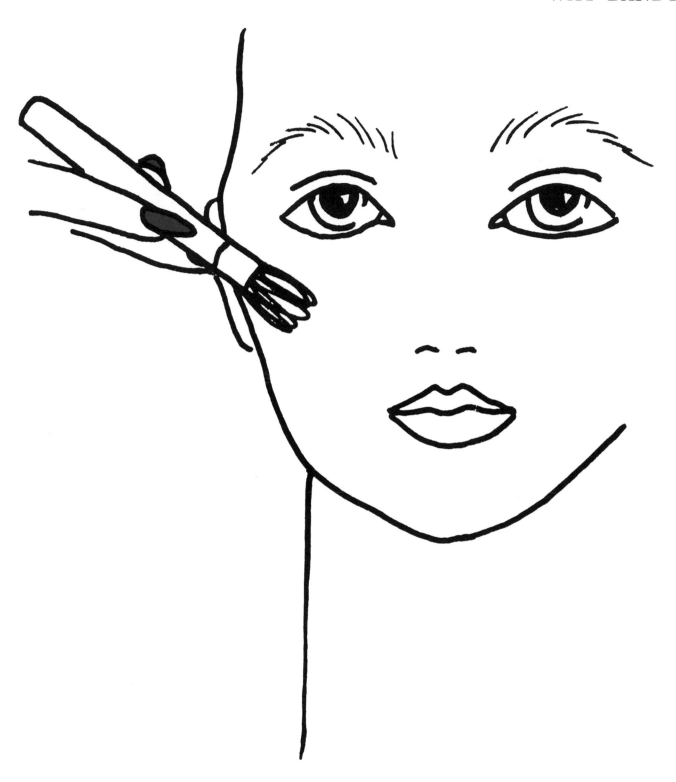

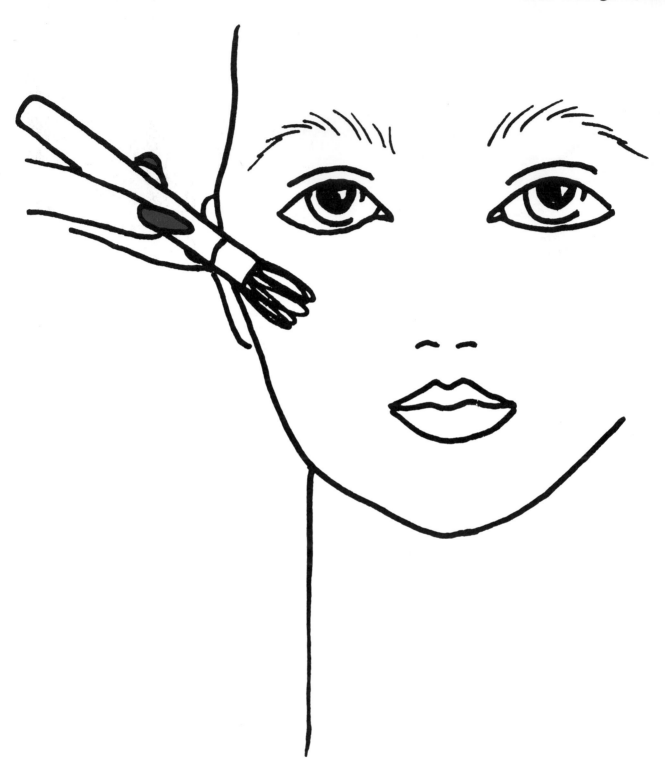

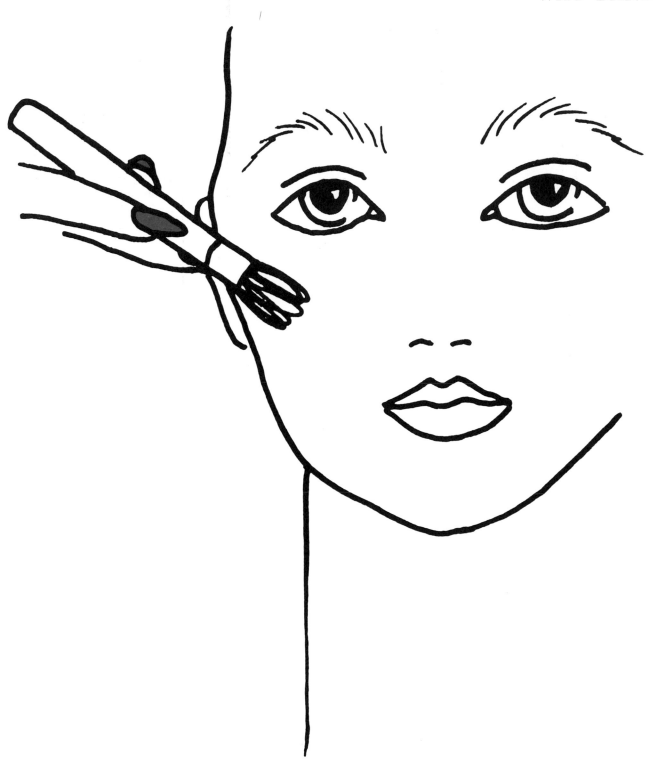

About the Author

WAY BANDY, a native of the American South, has been an artist all his life, specializing in the portraits of women.

After college and a few years spent as a teacher of American and English literature, he moved to New York City in 1967 to pursue a career in art. Sidetracked into the field of cosmetics by necessity—to pay the rent—Way discovered that he truly loved exaggerating and creating the illusion of facial beauty using cosmetics. From 1969 to 1971 he worked as Salon and Makeup Director for Lanvin-Charles of the Ritz. In 1972 Way began his current career as a free-lance face designer for fashion magazines such as *Vogue, Harper's Bazaar* and *Cosmopolitan*, where his work appears regularly. Way also designs for cosmetic advertising, television commercials, films and theatre.

The women on whose faces he has been privileged to work make a formidable list of international celebrity: Catherine Deneuve, Margaux Hemingway, Lauren Hutton, Diana Ross, Gloria Vanderbilt, Lee Radziwill, Barbra Streisand, Farrah Fawcett-Majors, Barbara Walters, Martha Mitchell (for her famous *New York* magazine make-over), Mary Tyler Moore, Cher, Polly Bergen, Dorothy Hamill, Jacqueline Bisset, Raquel Welch, Marisa Berenson, Iman, Billie Jean King, Martha Graham, Elizabeth Taylor, Claire Bloom and many others.